# The Shape of the Whole

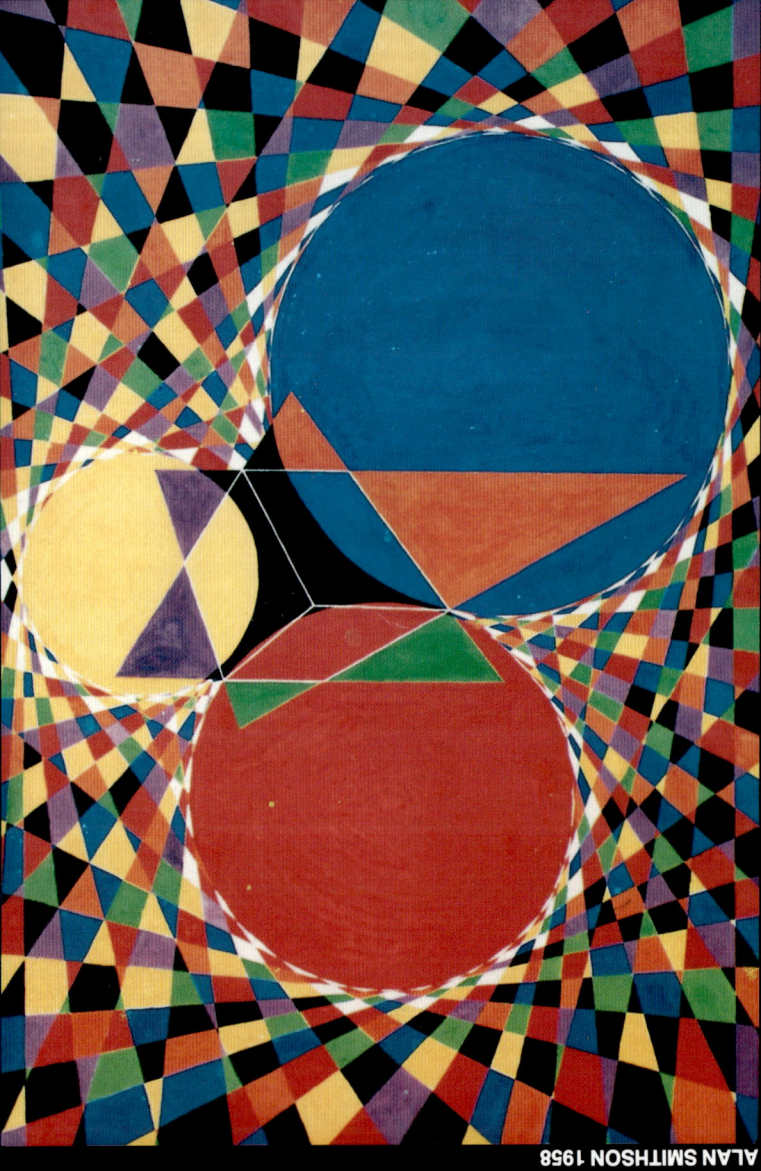

# The Shape of
# the Whole

## T.A. Smithson

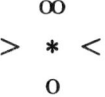

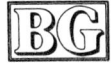

The Book Guild Ltd.
Sussex, England

The Book Guild Ltd.
25 High Street,
Lewes, Sussex.
First published 1990
© T.A. Smithson 1990
Set in Baskerville
Typesetting by Hawks Phototypesetters Ltd.,
Copthorne, West Sussex.
Printed in Great Britain by
Antony Rowe Ltd.,
Chippenham, Wiltshire.

British Library Cataloguing in Publication Data
Smithson, T.A. (Thomas Alan)
   The Shape of the Whole
   1. Philosophy
   I. Title
   100

ISBN 0 86332 508 4

*To*
*Ruth* **\*** *Jane*
*Mother*

Judge not according to the appearance, but judge righteous judgment.                    Jesus

To be, or not to be.                    Shakespeare

This same philosophy is a good horse in the stable, but an arrant jade on a journey.
                    Goldsmith

Quick now, here, now, always.                    Eliot

# CONTENTS

# INTRODUCTION

This volume presents some fundamental ideas in three different forms. There is a single painting, and two complementary written parts — a book and a paper, with appendices.

The painting at the beginning of the volume is a way of depicting the structure described in the written parts. You might regard it as an abstract icon, or a dynamic mandala — balanced but not symmetric. It stands without comment.

Part I consists of a book of twelve chapters. It sets out and explores the ideas, and incorporates aspects of my own experience. It touches on religious as well as philosophical matters, and in particular on the position of the person of Christ in relation to human life and understanding. It puts forward a view of the universe which questions many of our standard assumptions, and which I hope is coherent and positive without being rigidly dogmatic.

Part II is a paper which presents a more formal account of some of the principal ideas underlying the book. It is a kind of summary, but is better seen as a dual of Part I providing a complementary perspective. It extends the ideas and is more purely philosophical and abstract.

Appendix A gives a formal version of the Proof of Threeness discussed in Chapter 6. Appendix B gives an idea of what I mean by trinity and duality, and is worth glancing at before you read Chapters 6 and 7. Appendix C is a collection of 'seeds', germs of ideas which may spark off further ideas. Appendix D is a mathematical/metaphysical flight of fancy for those who may enjoy it.

I should like to acknowledge my debt to those who have been kind enough to read either or both parts of the volume, and have made helpful suggestions; in particular to Peter Baynes, Peter Bindley, Colin Dales, Noel Frieslich, Michael Le Mesurier, Margaret Richards, Geoffrey Rider, Ann Vaughan-Williams, Clive Wright, and especially to David Jackson and James Mark who have given generous and invaluable help. And to my wife Ruth for her patient and continual support during the time of gestation.

## Note on 'she/he'

There are few known female philosophers of note before our own times and so the feminine pronoun sounds odd when the reader knows that all or almost all the possible people in the context are male. I hope the growing number of distinguished women philosophers of our own day will therefore excuse my treating philosophers as 'he'. But there are other passages in this book where a bi-sexual form is desirable, and 'she/he' etc. would be clumsy.

The experimental solution I tried seemed too idiosyncratic and hard on the reader, and so eventually I chose in the book to use feminine forms in the odd-numbered chapters and masculine forms in the even-numbered (odd numbers are naturally male, and so a female pronoun in an odd-numbered chapter gives a bi-sexual meaning). Similarly in the paper feminine forms are used in the odd sections and masculine in the even. I hope this proves acceptable. It may be a useful reminder that meaning always depends on the relationship between word and context.

# PART ONE

# AS IF

## THE WORLD AS PRESENCE AND RELATIONSHIP

# CONTENTS

# PREFACE

This book is concerned with what is normally called metaphysics. It explores a perspective on life which is in many ways complementary to the normal academic one. The normal approach is to start with what we observe and experience, devise arguments for a metaphysical belief or for a philosophical position and show that the arguments are justified. The approach adopted here is to study the axiom that life is a unity. It is broadly personal, amateur, selective and intuitive, in contrast to the institutional, professional, exhaustive and formal approach of academic philosophy and theology.

The book arises out of a perception of conceptual integration which occurred in 1958 and resulted in the painting at the front of this volume. Attempts to discuss it at that time came to little. I put it aside for all practical purposes, working as a mathematician in a factory, in the central office of a large international firm, and in a small computer bureau (designing and writing a large amount of software), and recently as a software consultant on my own. Over the last decade I have begun to see that there are aspects which are worth trying to put into verbal form. The initial impetus came from Bryan Magee's 'Men of Ideas' programme on BBC TV, and this has been followed by a series of similar events which have led me to investigate the perception afresh.

The title is a phrase which occurs in the book a dozen times. It emphasizes that the way we speak about things always contains the element of 'asifness': whenever we talk in terms of a particular model (such as evolution) we are saying 'if you treat reality AS IF it is like this, you will interpret it correctly'. The theme of the book is the need to widen our sense of reality beyond the restricted AS IF's of science to reach the ultimate AS IF by which we orientate our lives.

The small list of references is provided to identify the sources of the few quotations, not to impress the reader with the breadth or otherwise of my reading. Any comment I make on the viewpoints of individuals does not aspire to be part of the professional dialogue. I have simply used their writings as jumping off points. In particular I have come back to Sir Karl Popper frequently because he seems to represent the best in modern scientific philosophy and I find his whole approach enjoyable and illuminating.

My own personal choices may surface from time to time, but they are not an essential part of the thesis. I am trying to set out what may for some be a fresh common approach to our situation, and to help to clear away some of the rubbish which centuries of thought have dumped at our door. The book covers a wide spectrum in a relatively small space. There is much more that could be said, but I hope that what is presented here forms an adequate first step.

Please do not feel obliged to read the whole book in order. Some parts may require fairly hard work, but the discussion is not a procedure like Euclid's in which each step depends on all the preceding ones, and skipping is certainly in order if you find yourself blocked. You may well omit parts of the more technical middle chapters on first reading. A glance at Appendix B should give you a quick idea of what I mean by 'trinity' and 'duality' before you read the written discussion. I am exploring a set of closely interrelated ideas merely in the order which was natural to me, and it is best if your feel free to follow your own nose through the whole thing rather than blindly follow my order — even if that does leave you with the burden of making your own decisions. The contents list and index offer help.

# 'AS IF' IN THE TEXT

The excerpts below comprise all the passages in which the phrase 'as if' occurs in the text. They offer a preliminary idea of the scope of the discussion.

## Chapter 2

When we look 'back' to the past all we can say is, 'The past looks to me to be AS IF such-and-such a model is valid.' Those words are simply the way in which we can best convey our sense of the truth as we utter them.

## Chapter 3

Once you have seen a mathematical truth it seems AS IF it has always been there. It is really an intuitive insight into the nature of necessity.

Some people try to objectify things like mathematical truths, making them into something hard 'out there' AS IF they 'exist' totally independently of us. The word 'exist' gives a false idea of their status.

Philosophers often discuss what is ultimately real, AS IF saying this or that could decide the matter. In fact what they are discussing is the way we think about everything.

## Chapter 5

There is a constant struggle, for instance, between Idealism and Realism, Intuitionism and Behaviourism, and so on. These are part of the continual debate which is fought out starting from different assumptions, and part of the game is to treat the assumptions AS IF they are absolutely true.

Philosophers spend a good deal of their time trying to score points off each other and dismissing each other's activities as irrelevant or meaningless. This must be taken seriously as part of the game at Level 2, but it is disastrous if it is taken to be at Level 1 — AS IF what is being sought is absolute truth.

## Chapter 10

To say that the problem of evil is solved does not help, because the offence of evil is always a real experience and to talk in terms of a solution AS IF to a mathematical problem would be quite wrong. But one can say that the formal metaphysical problem of evil is illusory.

Beginnings and ends belong to the dimension of finiteness and so have no ultimate reality in themselves. Any creation theory simply gives an AS IF answer to how we conceive of the beginnings of the universe in time.

## Chapter 11

The climate is created by a united determination which goes beyond the conscious level. When the time comes ideas spring into being, and it is AS IF they had been there all the time.

**Chapter 12**

All the old idealisms and realisms have been tried and have eventually been found wanting. Yet we still hanker after these solutions, AS IF they could ever provide a guarantee of Utopia.

But much of our talk is still in the language of historical and social processes, in terms of laws and forces and power. Science is spoken of AS IF it is wresting secrets from nature; politically minded people seek to reach positions of power and influence; the earth is still largely regarded as something to be exploited.

Scientists sometimes speak AS IF people's beliefs are illusions even though they work — for instance in healing. This kind of talk turns language on its head: the scientists themselves are under the illusion that facts have a reality which the beliefs do not.

# I

## IDEAS

The events of the last century have undermined all the old supposed certainties of religion and morality. Traditional values have been weakened, and many people have a sense of the seeming indifference of the universe to human existence. The evil in the world seems ineradicable. Much contemporary thought is deeply pessimistic. At the same time a great deal of practical activity is going on to arouse a sense of responsibility for the planet and to get people to live together in peace.

A vast amount of exploratory work has already been done by writers, artists and scientists to challenge the received ideas which pervade our thinking. Much of this was carried out around the turn of the century by the great modern pioneers of art and thought and science. There was a sea change in our intellectual perception of the world. Among the giants, in science there were Einstein, Heisenberg, Bohr; in art Cézanne, Picasso, Braque; in music Stravinsky, Ives, Bartok, Schoenberg; in philosophy Frege, Russell, Wittgenstein; in psychiatry Freud, Jung, Adler; in literature and drama Conrad, Joyce, Proust, Shaw, Ibsen. The list could be extended indefinitely in these and other fields.

Since then the wholly new areas of the cinema, radio, television and computing have appeared. At the same time the world has become one in a way which even half a century ago could barely have been imagined. In all these diverse changes there seems to be one underlying theme: there are no fixed explicit absolutes, we have to find the truth together as we live in relation to what we are.

The point was encapsulated by Moses long ago in the Second Commandment, which forbids the worship of graven images. Many people have still not recognized the simple truth underlying this law. A graven image is any finite structure which we treat as absolute. Fundamentalists of every kind are guilty of breaking the commandment, whether they worship the Bible, the Church, the Koran, the material world, scientific theories, Marxism, rationality, freedom, or equality. If we regard these simply as 'of great importance' we can relate them to other values, but to treat them as absolute is to elevate them to a position where it is they, rather than our living sense of what is right, that dictate our choices.

It is hard to learn this lesson. The loss of the old established values has for many led to an overriding feeling of disintegration. The power of the ancient ideas of absolutes and of hierarchy is still enormous. They have led to two terrible world wars, which have led in turn to disenchantment and then to the excesses of permissiveness in a search for new ways forward. There is now a reaction to that, but a simple return to the old values is not enough. If it continues to be accompanied by old ways of thinking it will be disastrous again.

This book is intended as a contribution towards getting things into better relationship. It is a hard and even risky task, because many of the old ideas are embedded in our habits of thought and they can easily well up into powerful emotions. At the same time modern languages, and perhaps especially English, have a freedom incorporated in them and a great many subtle concepts which were barely expressible in the ancient languages. One particularly valuable quality of English is the way it adjusts itself to the context in which words are used, so that the precision achieved is neither too great nor too little. It is also permeated by concepts such as fairness, freedom, courtesy, respect, consideration, imagination and tolerance. These are deeply embedded in the language and richly imbued with overtones of Prayer Book, Bible and Shakespeare and the great literary tradition which thrived on this foundation.

Such concepts have penetrated our background awareness to an extent which is barely realized. Many people now have a sense of what true freedom and justice means. They see it as a costly but not impossible goal, recognizing that it depends on each one of us, but is not some unattainable externally imposed ideal. It can be seen as going with the grain of reality, and acknowledging the truth, both conscious and unconscious, of what and where we are.

This is close to the heart of what Jesus taught and embodied. He came into a world which was rooted in the idea of a vertical hierarchy. While not ignoring the proper function of hierarchy he introduced a radical element which was primarily horizontal, emphasizing the essential equality of people as human beings. He brought this new comple-mentary element to bear on the excessive vertical emphasis of his times. He faces us with the challenge of unconditional love for our neighbour on the sole grounds that she is physically alongside us.

The old authoritarian ideas soon reasserted their hold — the ideas of absolute authority, absolute right, absolute truth which are in practice used to strengthen the position of those in power. As time went on these ideas were linked to the image of Jesus himself, the Church and the Bible. At the same time there has always been a core of true belief. It has taken twenty centuries of thought and suffering for people generally to begin to see through these graven images to the fact that the truth lies solely in a shared awareness of the truth.

☆        ☆        ☆

Many people recognize the need to transform the way we think about the world, along the lines pointed out to us by the great visionaries. One can have some sense of where they were pointing, but it is difficult to avoid being tricked by the habits of thought of a lifetime, and one finds oneself being caught out continually. Whatever I say here is conditioned by my upbringing and background, and is bound to be to that extent limited and incomplete and possibly sometimes misleading. It is one thing to feel that one has a clear conception in one's mind, and another to find the right words for it.

I do not propose to attempt anything exhaustive, partly because it is beyond my capacity, but especially because it would be a futile attempt to exclude everyone else. I shall make only a modest attempt to link with current literary and academic thought. I shall concentrate on only a few thinkers who seem to me representative figures about whom I have some knowledge. But I hope I can point to ways of reorientating our thinking which may get rid of some of the intellectual clutter which inhibits progress, so that we are free for the really important things. Too often in the past ideas have been used as tools of intellectual power, and they have resulted in enormous destruction. The idea that I am trying to develop may not seem to be an idea in the normal sense, since it results in no specific policies and no detailed explanations. It is simply a conception of our situation which may help towards a proper perspective on it and consequently a proper response.

We talk about mental structures, and this suggests the analogy of building. Building a house is a fairly simple process: we make a plan and put it into practice. We know the needs that have to be met, and we have a good idea of how they have been met in the past and what new possibilities there are. We finish up with a house which will suit some people better than others.

Even such a simple process can involve a good deal of interaction, especially when the buyer is having it made to his own specification. Unexpected situations can arise which could not have been foreseen. I had direct experience of this when we had a loft conversion done: the plans were all drawn up and the work itself actually started, and the carpenter suddenly realized that there was room for a window where the draughtsman had thought not. So the plan was completely re-drawn.

In the area of thought such re-thinking is the norm rather than the exception. We rarely have a simple concept which is then translated into reality. There is no visible product to be seen and judged. There is a continuous interaction between a whole set of concepts and the words used to express them and the judgments that we make about the world. A structure of thought is a set of interlocking judgments which is in continual flux, calling for a continuing flexible response.

The whole idea of 'putting ideas into practice' can be badly misleading. It suggests that first of all we have the idea, then we draw up detailed specifications, and these are then translated into reality. Although this is an adequate account of what happens externally, it gives the feeling of a one-way process which can be thoroughly mischievous in its effects. In fact there is a continuous interplay between the intractability of the material world and the awareness which is present in each individual involved.

Each task arises when a need is recognized. As we think about and discuss it, ideas arise out of the subconscious, and we select the one which we recognize as appropriate to the need. An idea has an abstract core whose nature is apprehended directly like a triangle or a circle: it is a living sense of the possibility of transformation, like Lancelot

Brown's 'capabilities'. Around that core it is malleable, and its realization grows and develops as it interacts with the material world through individual designers and managers and craftsmen.

In the case of building or manufacturing the stages of design, scheduling and execution tend to be fairly clearly defined. At the other end of the spectrum, in field of general ideas about how everything works, these stages remain conceptually distinct but they interact much more actively and intimately.

The understanding we are concerned with is not some theory which will 'explain' everything in detail to everyone. If we think about it it is at once clear that such a theory is impossible to achieve. Any theory has to be expressed in words or diagrams or examples, and the more comprehensive and complex the theory the longer it will take to express fully. As each element of the theory is expressed it must be related to every other element so far, and one can reach a point where more questions are being generated about preceding elements than there are answers coming in.

The only way to get around this problem is recognize the whole theory as a unity by a direct act of intuition. This is a frequent and normal experience for the student as her knowledge and understanding grows. When it happens for someone like Einstein at the frontiers of science, it is experienced as a moment of illumination of particular significance because it marks a stage not only in her own progress but in that of everyone. Apart from its comprehensiveness and practical significance, however, the experience of both the student and Einstein is essentially the same.

At points like these a special link is forged between inner and outer reality. Such moments should be neither undervalued nor overvalued, but simply seen as stages which are experienced as specially significant. They are points at which the possibilities made available by a vast array of apparently trivial choices are focused in a particular concrete situation, and new vistas are opened up. Moments of discovery, moments of heroism, moments of love are all essentially alike. They are specially transcendent moments in which a particular environment is so caught up and penetrated by the living truth that it becomes a secure anchor point tethering the shifting framework of space and time to reality.

'Ordinary' people often regard such experiences as beyond their conception. That is because they have been educated into thinking that the important things only happen at the level of an Einstein. Such a view unjustly diminishes each person and attempts to devalue what is going on inside her. Every experience which leads us to our own personal flash of insight, at whatever level, is essentially of the same kind. Every time we say yes to the truth in the most 'minor' decision we open the way to such experiences.

Understanding once formulated runs the immediate risk of becoming a graven image. As soon as one has found something there is a temptation to hang onto it as one's own. The most damaging graven images are fixed conceptions of the world — *idées fixes* — which are logical extensions of a single idea expressed in absolute external form. Such noble images are to be treated with respect: they embody the work and striving of people who were seeking the truth. We 'worship' a graven image only when we treat it as absolute, by allowing it to determine our judgments automatically.

*Idées fixes* are like the walled cities which men used to

build in order to make possible a peaceful and civilized life. All great social structures tend to rely on them in large measure. They make rules and build mental walls and tell people, 'You must adhere to the rules and stay inside the walls, otherwise you will weaken the city and destroy yourself. We will take the strongest measures against you if you do not conform, and if you persist we shall be forced to cast you out.' The irony of this is that as soon as a visionary rebel who is aware of the true good of the city is cast out, this destroys the unity at which the rules were aimed. Socrates and Jesus experienced this paradox in all its depth.

That is true of the great philosophies as well. These are great mental edifices before which we stand in awe at the sensitivity and subtlety with which the interrelationships between different aspects are explored. They offer great intellectual riches to the students of each new generation. But like the civilizations with which they are closely linked there is always the danger that they will reach a point at which the whole edifice no longer tolerates interaction. It becomes fossilized and attempts to dominate creative individuals by claiming absolute authority.

Plato provides a profound example of this. When at school I studied his *Apology of Socrates* and was captivated and wholly won over by Socrates himself. But I follow Sir Karl Popper in feeling that Plato, Socrates's star pupil who thought and wrote so beautifully and brilliantly, contrived nevertheless to lead us astray in fundamental ways. A brief discussion of two aspects of Plato's thought may help to illustrate what I am getting at, and introduce a way of thinking that I shall be developing.

One source of trouble can be found in his concept of the Forms (goodness, truth, and so on), which are among the most celebrated of his ideas. He seems to treat them as absolutes existing independently of our normal experience. While he may himself have recognized the limits to the way in which the concept is to be used, it has encouraged a deeply rooted habit of thought which locates abstract entities beyond the world, and sees them as providing the ideal model which is then to be copied into some material embodiment. This way of thinking is endemic to our culture.

He was right in seeing that reality is inward. He comes somewhere near the truth in suggesting that appearances are a sort of shadow of reality, though it is better to call them a presentation since a shadow is so much more elusive than our personal experience. He is right to see ideas such as circles and triangles as being very pure concepts which provide the most basic common ground when we discuss and relate to the physical world. He is right to say that a clear understanding of these Forms and their properties is an invaluable aid to a true insight into reality.

He leads us astray however if we infer that there exists a Form of absolute goodness/beauty/truth which must be *applied* to the situation we are discussing. His ideas actually gave rise among the later Christian Platonists to arguments about whether God himself was subordinate to the Forms. Viewed in this way they become graven images of a very far-reaching sort.

The idea of Forms has a pre-packed quality. It encourages the idea that there is a predefined Form for each situation. This inherently ignores one of the basic facts about each situation, namely its newness. There are always areas of ignorance which we can do nothing about: they are an essential part of the way the moment is presented to us. The Form must take into account this element of newness and unknownness, but since the Forms are exemplified by things like circles and straight lines it is easy to overlook the need to incorporate these elements.

To use the language of Forms properly, we need to recognize that the absolute Form of Good is the Form which allows presence to fill the moment of decision in such a way that known and unknown, past and future, inner and outer are brought into wholeness, in full relationship with the truth of all other person-moments. To have a comprehensive conception of the Form of Good we have to see it as full openness to what is required in the situation, without preconceptions: the only acceptable preconception is that the choice is not predetermined. Out of this openness arises the simple choice of 'Yes' or 'No' immediately we recognize both moment and truth.

All subsidiary Forms such as beauty and truth and justice are simply attempts to be more specific, since they imply that the particular category is more relevant to the situation than the others. This may or may not be so. The choice of the appropriate category is the basic decision. If we take it for granted that a particular Form is appropriate we prejudge the whole issue. A common example of such an abuse of subsidiary Forms is to take it for granted that the scientific approach is automatically appropriate. We bow down to a graven image instead of placing it alongside others in our pantheon of gods who are present but are not absolute.

Any act of understanding is a matter of interpretation, and interpretation is closely linked with hidden hints in the language. Plato's idea of pre-existent Forms like immovable constellations in the world of the mind can easily lead to a wrong conception of what is right. He talks about the Forms being timeless, and this can give one the idea that in a given situation there is an exact abstract model of what we have to do in order to realize the Good. That is misleading. But there is also a sense in which he is right to use the word. If it helps us to see that there is a possible absolute rightness in the way we meet a situation, and that it is always the same in being absolute whatever its *outward* form, the word 'timeless' is completely right.

The other major weakness one is aware of in Plato is his
élitism, which reveals a Gnostic and authoritarian
tendency. He assumes that he knows best, and wants to
impose his regime: he seeks to compel people to accept his
ideas because the Forms are good for them. It is hardly
surprising that his attempt to put his ideas into practice in
Syracuse was a failure: he would appear as someone coming
along with all the answers, and forgetting the need for the
people involved to want them.

It is of course easy to look back and see how his ideas
have been misunderstood and have misled people. He had
to work with the language and ideas available at the time,
and his achievement within that constraint in a small and
limited civilization is quite unparalleled. He says himself
that he is talking in similes, and these are valid provided we
interpret them rightly. For example he says in *The Republic*,
'In my opinion, for what it is worth, the final thing to be
perceived in the intelligible realm, and perceived only with
difficulty, is the absolute form of Good; once seen, it is
inferred to be responsible for everything right and good.
Anyone who is going to act rationally either in public or in
private must perceive it.' If we understand 'the form of
Good' as his way of saying 'what is right for the whole' this
is finely stated, and with humility.

Plato's thought may have led to errors along the lines
indicated, but his method has been immensely productive
and creative. Many features of his thought remain perma-
nently valid. It has mingled fruitfully with Christian
dialectics, and has encouraged the disinterested search for
truth and values. It has provided a strong foundation for
the structures built by thinkers such as Augustine, Thomas
Aquinas and Hegel. Any such structure, however, is
developed in relation to its epoch. Each model only remains
valid with limits, and as new situations are met strains are
bound to arise between any explicitly formulated model and

reality. We have to recognize the points at which we move outside the bounds of the model into regions where it is no longer wholly valid.

To some extent we have to accept such a unified system warts and all. Each is a ladder like Wittgenstein's for people to climb up at the stage they are at, and is not necessarily fit to be used as it stands for the next stage. Civilizations build the first storey on the ground; when they get to the first floor each uses its own ladder consisting of some system of thought which unifies their perception of their situation. But each ladder will only reach to a limited height, and many people find the ladders of other cultures are of no help even if they are longer.

To extend upwards from the base of existing cultures and link them all so that there is general access we need something different. It must be something which all of us can use, which can go virtually as high as we need, and which incorporates the whole experience of the past. Instead of a ladder we need a crane, which can cover the whole building from top to bottom, and can link outside and inside. A crane is a response to a real need, and the idea of it arises out of a fresh approach using all the relevant experience and techniques that are available. Those are the lines we need to work on, but the venture has to be a co-operative one aimed at linking many other ways of viewing what I am discussing here. My own offering is to suggest some ideas for a metaphysical crane, which like the ladder can be dispensed with when it has served its purpose.

# 2

## THE STRUCTURE OF REALITY

In this chapter I propose to sketch the outline of a metaphysical conception of the world in as simple terms as I can. The conception will be developed in later chapters; here I shall concentrate on the relevance of the conception to the problem of evil, and shall discuss two examples of evil as experienced in reality.

The subtitle of this book is *The World as Presence and Relationship*. The idea underlying this phrase is that reality is a whole within which all our experiences are related. A word which brings us somewhere near to the nature of this total reality is 'spirit'. It is an infinity of infinities within which our finite experiences interact with each other. Simultaneously it is a oneness which lies at the heart of all subordinate onenesses.

Discussing numbers in his late writings Kierkegaard says: 'In the world of sense one adds up, and it becomes a large number, in the world of spirit one adds up and the large number vanishes as in a conjuring trick.' Spirit is awareness. There is no difference in kind between you and me and him and her in being aware of ourselves being aware. Size and numbers and position make no difference to that: they belong to the dimension of relationship, not of awareness.

The oneness and indivisibility of awareness is something we can each recognize. We are all aware that we are all aware, and this means that what we have in common is this common awareness of our situation. The consciousnesses are separate, with separate points of view, and the awareness is the same. Elitists are constantly in danger of ignoring this truth, but they cannot honestly deny that the person they despise is aware like themselves of the 'thisness' of the situation in which they meet. Our modes of being are different, but the reality dwelling in us all is the same. It is not easy to give it a name because we are talking of the whole, and the whole is ultimately ineffable. At various times we may use the words spirit, or love, or truth, or beauty, or presence, or reality, or God.

This awareness is experienced as a recognition of the truth of where we are. At each moment we have the choice of saying yes or no to our recognition. For those who wish to use the language of 'sin', this is the only point at which sin occurs: sin has nothing to do directly with external acts. For those who dislike that terminology, the idea of a 'sense of rightness' can be used in referring to the same absolute choice. If we say no we cut our awareness off from reality. Having done this we are likely to continue to shy away. We can only face up to reality again if we recognize and accept the cost we have left others to carry. We are all completely vulnerable to each other's choices. Each choice is an absolute yes/no which is a critical determinant of the feel and shape of the whole.

The external direction of the truth of our situation cannot be predicted automatically. There are many pointers which help us to focus our attention in making a hard decision, but no generalization is possible such as 'choose the new' or 'choose the old'. For each of us the decision has to be 'my own', because only 'I' am in the position where it can be made. 'I' have to treat it as open right up to the point at which it is taken. At the same time 'my own' has to involve 'your own' because the situation involves you simultaneously, and the truth lies in our shared awareness of the whole.

The story of the widow's mite is a constant reminder that we can have no idea of the depth or significance of what is going on inside the most apparently ordinary or 'worthless' person. Every moment of choice is of equal worth in the eternal dimension, and from that point of view comparisons are irrelevant: the most trivial decision which says 'yes' to the truth potentially outweighs the most momentous 'no', since 'yes' is alive and 'no' is dead. The greatest writers point up this truth in their works again and again.

We experience the complementary aspects of the world as inner and outer, past and future, known and unknown, actual and potential. The relationships between these are in a state of continual flux, and as things are filled out there are aspects of the structure which are (to our eyes) thrown out of balance by 'wrong' choices. Wrong choices are experienced as disorders in the external world and as corresponding personal pain in the inner world. The necessary relationship between inner and outer incorporates the 'wrong' choice and makes it part of the structure. This leads to the emergence of situations where opportunities are created for the 'imbalance' to be healed: right choices at these points, requiring costly openness to whatever is required, can embrace and transform the emptiness of the wrong choice.

One way of visualizing this is to picture the physical world as a kind of four-dimensional sculpture in space-time. From this point of view it consists of a vast array of person-moments, points at the intersection of inner and outer, at each of which there is the possibility of wholeness entering. Each of us is aware of the freedom to say yes or no to our own sense of integrity in the moment of choice. If we take light as an analogue of wholeness, the colour and quality and intensity of the light depend on our situation and we can do nothing about them, but we have complete freedom about saying yes or no to whether we let the light through.

This is where the possibility of meaning lies. If we say yes, a moment of meaning is built into the body of the world and reaches out to link with all other such moments. If we say no, it leaves a wound in the flesh of the world at that moment which can only be healed by some other yes.

We habitually conceive of the world as stretching back in time, with successive events depending causally on each other. That is a good model for many purposes, but one must always keep in mind that it *is* a model — a way of communicating an idea of underlying reality. While it may be close to reality in certain respects, it always reduces it to something less, and there may well be aspects which are completely wrong.

It is easy to slip into the trap of thinking that the past is objectively there, and that it has generated everything that follows. That is a useful way of thinking for some purposes, but it is just as true, and much truer from the point of view of an overall understanding, to say that as we make decisions we continually create both the past and the future simultaneously. The past is simply one particular aspect of the present.

This is hard to accept, because Darwinian ideas and ideas about the direction of time are so firmly entrenched. We 'know' that early humans evolved slowly out of the animal kingdom, with all its brutishness, and had to struggle for existence against the elements and against their neighbour. But we are trying to conceive of what 'really' happened by setting up our idea of the past, and saying, 'Everything I find fits in with my idea, and so that is what really happened.' That is certainly appropriate for practical and scientific purposes, but reality is essentially what we are aware of as being true in the present. When we look 'back' to the past all we can say is, 'The past looks to me to be AS IF such-and-such a model is valid.' Those words are simply the way in which we can best convey our sense of the truth as we utter them.

If we ask the question, 'Did a man on August 29th 9018 BC, at grid reference . . . in the middle of Africa, strike his brother at 10.01 am and kill him?' there may not be a yes/no answer to that question even in principle. We have first of all to ask whether it is permissible and meaningful to ask the question. The questions that we ask determine the answers that we are going to get, and so they have to be the right ones.

We have to make the decision that it is right to ask the question now and begin to seek an answer. Perhaps we should be doing something entirely different. Asking questions and discussing the answers is a real activity. It takes place in real people in the real world and so it is an area in which we are making choices which involve awareness of what is right — not in a 'moralistic' sense, but in the sense of our hunch at the deepest level about what is needed.

Assuming it is appropriate to ask it, the question can be answered in principle as truthfully as any other question of historical fact. We can seek out evidence, we can use theories which we have good reason to believe are sound, we can discuss it all with everyone who we think could help. These discussions will all assume the structures of time and place and words and concepts and human beings.

How far we are prepared to go depends primarily on two things: how much we ourselves feel in our bones that it matters, and how certain we think we need to be. We may be free to go on and on, depending on our circumstances and resources. We may decide we have no hope of knowing one way or another. We may be asked to commit ourselves before we feel ready, and we will have to decide whether this is a temptation or a challenge. We may come to a point where we are so certain within ourselves that we are prepared to commit ourselves to a definite answer which we are willing to defend against all comers.

But we will never be able to answer yes or no with absolute objectivity, even though we may reach an inner sense of complete conviction. All we will have is a growing confidence which arises out of living with the question, together with an authority which goes hand in hand with this, but which is entirely dependent on the integrity with which we pursue the quest. Moreover that integrity involves not only our honesty with ourselves, but also the way in which we handle offers of help. Integrity requires us to recognize the point at which we need to accept help from others.

Facts are the product of choices, and historical facts are the products of historians' judgments both on their correctness and their relevance. A fact in a written history is the expression of the writer's judgment in the form of a verbal account. But our thinking is easily dominated by simplistic ideas about historical facts as something independent of human choice. This can lead us either to attribute injustice to the universe or to think that there is some ultimate division between good and evil or between spirit and matter. Although the scientific spirit is a major manifestation of true awareness it simply does not concern itself with the way in which human choice relates to fact. It concerns itself with the connections in the observable world, but not with the unique event in itself. It may have plenty to say about the structure of the smallpox virus and the opposing vaccine, but it has nothing to say about precisely why Saida has smallpox now. That is a fact whose significance and reason can only be found in its relationship to the whole pattern of choice.

The picture I am suggesting is that the world as we experience it is the precise product of human choice, and that the core of each choice lies completely hidden within each person. It lies at the point where he assents to or denies his recognition of the true choice, where he chooses whether to trust his awareness of the truth. The fact of particular noes is presented to us as the experience of evil. The noes create a distortion of the balance between inner and outer worlds. What we experience is the proper and exact reflection of this distortion.

This conception provides a metaphysical resolution of the problem of evil. We can interpret evil as the necessary outcome of negative choices at particular moments, and this frees us from the dualistic idea of a Devil or an evil deity or an absolute split between mind and body. It permits a non-dualistic picture of creation as arising out of nothingness in a way which takes nothingness seriously. We can see reality as presenting us all with experiences which respect nothingness and maintain continuity and consistency. This may be difficult to imagine, but the idea itself is not difficult to conceive. Chapter 7 gives some hints on the way we can think of it as working.

Something similar to this picture has been put forward in the past, explaining evil as a kind of hole in creation. This is inadequate if it leads to an easy optimism which disregards the reality of evil as we encounter it. We have to take care not to explain away evil.

The idea has value primarily on the metaphysical level. It points to the fact that evil is necessary but in no sense ultimate. Evil is necessary because the moment when a person says no, as an act of deliberate choice against his true judgment, must immediately be built into the truth of the new state of affairs. Each such rejection is an emptiness, a denial of awareness and a shirking of responsibility, and it must be reflected precisely in the interrelationship between internal and external phenomena. An emptiness in the Choice World is expressed as a mismatch between the inner and outer worlds. This is what we experience as evil, and it confronts us with the reality of what has to be resolved, in terms which are meaningful if we read them rightly.

The metaphysical danger of regarding evil as ultimate is that it gives us an excuse for avoiding the responsibility that we face in each moment. We can blame 'the Devil' for leading us astray, and since he is thought of as operating at the divine level we can say 'I couldn't help it'. We can also identify the Devil with some enemy, and delude ourselves that by destroying the enemy we will destroy the Devil. In truth the evil we experience is the presentation of the disharmony of humanity as it relates to us, and the first thing to learn is that each of us bears an equal responsibility to face up to that — *alongside* any human enemy we may happen to have.

In the light of this picture we can consider two particular kinds of evil which a lot of people have trouble with intellectually:

1. Pain which the sufferer cannot cope with;
2. Natural disasters which appear to be uncon-nected with human actions.

The thought nags away at the back of our minds that these things would happen whatever choices were made. This may lead us to feel that there is something inherently unjust about them which implies an absolute indifference on the part of the universe.

We can widen the first example to include all those who find life too much for them to bear. Any simple explanation would be intolerably glib. The scandal is not only something for the person himself to bear, but for us to take into ourselves. To pretend there is no scandal is to avoid sharing the cost. At the same time a sense of the wholeness of things requires us to conceive that it was absolutely necessary that it should happen. One can have the idea that it is a matter of cosmic grief that it is necessary. There is a terrifying logic involved: the necessity must arise because of the constraints within which the world comes into being.

To the question, 'Why this person at this time in this particularly dreadful way?' there is only the reply, 'Because whatever our limited perception of the situation may be, that was the proper presentation of the truth of the pattern of choices as it related to that person at that time in that particular situation.' Sometimes the connection will seem obvious, but much more often it will be deeply hidden and will have little to do with the ordinary understanding and the 'rights of the case'. Part of the significance of what happens is that we ourselves are aware of the scandal and have to become involved. If we tried to go into all the details of why it was proper we should go on indefinitely: the process can only come to an end in an immediate sense that it was right when every detail is fully taken into account. To recognize that is to be aware that it was what the whole configuration required. But to talk about it in these terms in a particular case is hardly possible.

We can conceive that there is a logic — along the lines of the logic of a play or a piece of music or painting or poetry — which must be followed if creation is to take place without cheating. What happens is absolutely precisely linked to the configuration of the Choice World. This resembles Einstein's conception of the physical universe: the current configuration of mass is precisely linked to the curvature of space, so that the way things are now is directly related to the geometry of the way things develop.

Einstein's theory is a physical, 'single' version of the idea of the ultimate interdependence of form and content, reflecting the universal principles of balance and unity. Concepts like these, general as they are, are abstractions which we make from what has already happened. They can help us to realize that there is a form to be recognized in what happens, and so sense how this applies in our situation now.

In the second case, the earthquake, we are scandalized by

its arbitrariness. There seems to be nothing in common between the people who die or suffer in the earthquake except that they are in the same place at the same time. But the earthquake too is a response to persons' choices, to what one might call the total spiritual state: it is simply that the connection with the Choice World is much more hidden. The earthquake involves much longer time spans, and is more intimately linked not only with what has happened but with what will happen in persons' minds as a result of it. It provides an immediate challenge for the rescuers, it makes people remember the fragility of life, it spurs on investigation into the ways in which people can be warned of impending catastrophe, it prompts us to ask the question we have asked. None of these justifies the event in itself, but there is nothing arbitrary about it: we can think of it as a 'decision by reality' which is made in the light of all the implications and constraints.

People are there when the earthquake happens because there is an imperfect relationship between them and the environment. It is not the fault of those particular people, or at least not solely so: it is an expression of the state of the whole. We tend to think that earthquakes 'are bound to happen' and that people 'are bound to be killed'. In our present state these are valid statements, so long as we recognize that they are based on the state of the Choice World *as it is*. As individuals we cannot do anything about it, but it is vital to recognize that there is no logical connection between the apparent arbitrariness of such events and the belief that they are arbitrary in an ultimate sense. If we think that there is we undermine our ultimate values with false logic, and surrender our sense of responsibility to fatalism.

There is one superficial point of difference between earthquakes and events such as air crashes. Both of them involve many people who happen to be in the same environment at the same time. Something happens which renders the environment incapable of tolerating human life. But the earthquake is totally beyond man's control, while the air crash is in most cases the result of human error. However the difference is not as great as we imagine. People, in the West particularly, are always looking for close associations between human choice and actual events. This is the area in which there are the most obvious rewards, which can be grasped immediately. It is the area in which scientific investigation operates with greatest effect. But there are deeper processes going on, and these always bring us back to the whole situation.

It may not be easy to see that such events are much magnified versions of tragedies that we are aware of as happening all the time. But scale does matter to some extent, and we might ask, if the whole of the earth were to be destroyed, how could that be justified?

If that did happen there would be nobody to justify it to, while until it does there is no need to justify it. We have to face the fact that it is a possibility, since people cannot be forced to say yes, and if the configuration of yeses and noes is such that that is the right thing to happen, it will happen. It is a challenge to us to look the unthinkable in the face, and to realize that everything depends on each of us. It may help us to concentrate our minds on transforming life so that the unthinkable cannot become the right thing to happen. The real danger lies in loss of nerve, from which the West has suffered deeply in this century. Optimism and pessimism are equally out of place: what is needed is a recognition of the nature of our situation and a determination to respond to it as openly as we can.

# 3

## FINITE AND INFINITE

It is worth trying to achieve a general perspective on the status of philosophy and particular philosophies. There is a vast spectrum of these ranging in a great arc from Materialism to Idealism and back again, and all of them draw attention to facets of experience which have to be taken into account.

Particular philosophies can be regarded as two-dimensional diagrams of reality. Each one may contain many different cross-sections, covering the whole of 'reality' with a coarse or a fine grid of diagrams, but each does so from an established viewpoint. Each starts from some basic presupposition about the fundamental nature of reality, and as soon as this is expressed in words and arguments it imposes restrictions and limitations. In the regions of reality where the plane of the cross-section coincides with the natural grain we will get a very accurate representation of reality, but in the regions where the grain is at right-angles to the plane the picture will be totally uninformative. It will indeed be positively misleading, since it will in effect imply that a whole dimension simply does not exist.

What is true of philosophies is also true of persons. Each person is tied to her own perspective, and her view of the world is analogous to the planes of the philosophic diagrams. There are regions of reality which are known — *ie*. the plane goes with the grain — and there are regions of ignorance where the grain is at right angles.

For a fully adequate representation of reality we need something analogous to a three-dimensional model. In the case of philosophy the model is built up of words and ideas. Logical arguments only apply within parallel planes; there is no way for instance that an argument on a subjective level can be linked purely logically to an argument on an objective level. The attempt to do this leads to all kinds of paradoxes and mental confusions. So what we are looking for is a way of conceiving of the structure of the whole of reality, taking full account of the rightness and detail of the two-dimensional diagrams, but going beyond these so that we have a sense of them 'in the round'.

It is in this respect that Wittgenstein is such an exceptional thinker. After solving (as he believed) all the purely formal problems of philosophy in the *Tractatus*, by splitting the conceptual domain of language into what can be said and what cannot be said, he realized that this was all in the plane of pure theory. The Achilles' heel of his approach was that he was unable to supply a single example of an 'atomic fact': in other words he could not tether his theory to reality. So he went off and pondered further, and reached a view which was at right angles to his earlier view, set out in his *Philosophical Investigations*. It was concerned with what happens in real life, the language and other games that people play.

The two approaches are beautifully complementary, gaining in significance because they are both works by the same person. There is no point in asking which is right in absolute terms: the simple answer is that it depends on which face of reality we need to deal with at the moment. There is probably no one who has absorbed the intellectual tension between complementary ways of looking at things so deeply into himself. By taking it into his own life he was going far deeper than any monist thinker can get, and showing that the link between viewpoints and the resolution of paradoxes can only be achieved within the consciousness of a human being who is prepared to accept the personal cost. The perennial weakness of monism is that, even though superficially it is formally valid in the plane of the *Tractatus*, it does not face up to the tension and the reality of the concrete situation.

This aspect of theoretical knowledge is something I found very difficult when younger. One can be aware of the formal validity of an argument, but it is too easy to assume that it can be expressed directly. If one is not careful one ends up with platitudes. Everything collapses into a dull uniformity because one is aware of an empty structure which has no life. It is completely unrelated to reality and so can seem pointless. I encountered this disillusioning experience when studying mathematics at university, and something similar is recorded by Bertrand Russell. He observed that mathematics ceased to be interesting to him when he came to see it as one immense tautology, which could be directly apparent as such to a superhuman mind.

One can jump to this conclusion when looking at a statement like '$2 + 2 = 4$' which once absorbed becomes part of one's assumptions: it is experienced as obvious. The statement provides a means of looking at the same set of events in two different ways which are in one particular respect (the mathematical) exactly related. It is a way of saying that you can look at any set of four things as two pairs: you can choose the way in which you look at them. The corollary of this is that if you know you have two pairs of things, you know immediately (without going through the operation of actually counting) that you have four things. So if I tell you I have put two oranges in a bag, and then another two, and *if* I can assume that you know that $2 + 2 = 4$, then I can assume that you know that there are four oranges in the bag.

But it is possible that you do not know that $2+2=4$, and in that case my assumption about your knowledge will be wrong. You may only be able to interpret the oranges in the bag as two pairs of oranges. So while I have two ways of looking at the final result, and can not only choose which one to use but can be aware of their necessary relationship, you have only one way. By making us aware of such relationships mathematics enlarges our awareness of the world: it enables us to hold different viewpoints simultaneously in our mind.

When teaching mathematics I found it hard to remember learning what I knew. Once you have seen a mathematical truth it seems as if it has always been there. It is really an intuitive insight into the nature of necessity, a perception of truth in the formal plane, a sense of rightness about our concepts which we take for granted in our intercourse. We easily forget that the activity of linking the concepts through language and diagrams takes place in time and requires attention like any other process. Moreover even '$2+2=4$' is only true within a defined set of axioms, and it is of great interest to find what the minimum set of axioms is. And it is of endless interest to investigate, extend and simplify the external presentation of the complex self-consistent structure of mathematics.

Some people try to objectify things like mathematical truths, making them into something hard 'out there' as if they 'exist' totally independently of us. The word 'exist' gives a false idea of their status. If we replace it by 'hold good if the axioms are satisfied' we are more likely to avoid the metaphysical error. It is a subtle point. A mathematical truth formulates a necessary connection. It says, 'if you assume this collection of facts and this structure, then you can assume this second collection of facts'. When it has been completely absorbed by a person, it becomes an internalized immediate knowledge which can unify different aspects of our experience if it is recognized to apply. It is not a thing in itself: the formula is a way in which we express our knowledge of a particular aspect of necessity. We choose to work on a particular formula because we recognize that our knowledge of necessity in that area is inadequate. This choice is made in the real world in real time. The formulas we happen to be taught are therefore products of the historical process which we have actually perceived and judged to be significant unities: they are just as much our creations as they are 'objective truths'. They are unavoidably true, but that only matters if they are also significant.

This tendency to objectify is a general characteristic of much of Western thought, and it extends to both objects and concepts. We normally treat these as 'real' things having a free-standing existence of their own. There is little harm in this except for our overall sense of what is going on. The danger lies in jumping from 'for all appropriate practical purposes' to 'for all purposes', and it is quite fundamental to the way we understand the world. Every object or concept can be treated as 'objectively real' only within a bounded domain. If we try to extend its absoluteness beyond that domain we deny the need to relate it to everything else. In the last resort, though for practical purposes objects and concepts exist and have the properties we analyse and discuss, they are simply particular experiences through which we experience a single reality.

The eighteenth century philosopher Berkeley was extremely clear on this point, though many people have still managed to misunderstand what he said, even those purporting to be his spokesmen. His beautifully written work *Three Dialogues between Hylas and Philonous* puts his view with crystal clarity. I found it strange that in the introduction in my edition, probably written early in this century, the editor Thomas McCormack of Illinois regards a key passage as having been the one passage which 'leaves his achievement of a perfect spiritual monism incomplete'. The same passage had in 1871 been considered by Professor Fraser to be the most remarkable in the dialogues.

Hylas, arguing for a materialist view, says: 'Notwithstanding all you have said, to me it seems that, according to your own way of thinking, and in consequence of your own principles, it should follow that *you* are only a system of floating ideas, without any substance to support them.' Philonous the philosopher, speaking for Berkeley, replies: 'How often must I repeat, that I know or am conscious of my own being; and that I *myself* am not my ideas, but somewhat else, a thinking, active principle that perceives, knows, wills and operates about ideas.'

Berkeley refers to objects too as 'ideas', since he regards all phenomena as ultimately 'mental'. He uses the words 'mental' and 'mind' in the widest possible sense, embracing our whole experience as persons — our thoughts and feelings and our whole sense of ourselves. However McCormack thinks that Berkeley is talking about the ego. He says in criticism 'both Hylas and Hume have been upheld by modern scientific psychology in their rejection of an ego-identity.' It is certainly true that any concept of the I in terms of Berkeley's temperament, background, knowledge, abilities and so on would not be adequate. But this is not what Berkeley is talking about. He is talking about the living awareness within himself which is stretching out to meet the *same* awareness within Hylas and within all those who seek to understand the metaphysical truth. That is ultimately where the validity of his argument lies, and the whole book is simply a record of his willingness to lay open this awareness to the deepest possible scrutiny, trusting that it is strong enough to face every intellectual test.

There is a way of picturing the kind of conception which Berkeley was arguing for. It can be set out in the form of a cross as follows:

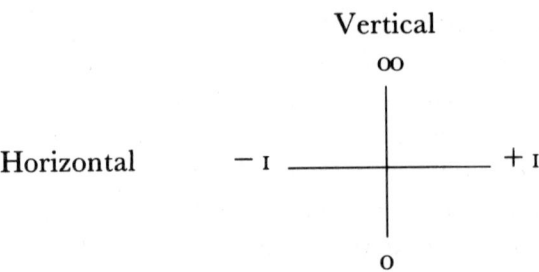

We can interpret this diagram as representing the fundamental categories of our experience. There are two fundamentally orthogonal categories, represented by the vertical line and the horizontal line. The vertical line represents the eternal, infinite, absolute categories. At the top is the infinite reality of self-awareness; at the bottom the zero necessity of self-consistency. The horizontal line represents the temporal, finite, relative categories of 'actual' phenomena, which take the two basic forms of internal and external.

The whole pattern represents the basic structure of creation as consisting of the single external world ($+1$) of objects balancing and reflecting the multiple internal world ($-1$) of subjects (persons). Both of these worlds are experienced as finite: they embody relationships which are poised between the poles of infinite awareness and nothingness. These finite worlds involve the dimension of time as well as space, and we can regard the basic unit in both as the *event*, which has concurrent internal and external aspects.

We can take the mathematical analogy further. If we multiply infinity by zero we can get any value we like by defining the process of multiplication as we choose. So on the face of it both internal phenomena and external phenomena are arbitrary. But the phrase used was 'as we choose'. It is choice which determines the relationship between inner and outer events. We as individuals choose to say yes or no, and our experience faces us with the proper response to our choices. The actual configuration which we experience presents us with the balance between inner and outer which truly reflects the pattern of our choices.

The diagram does not show the categories themselves, but symbols for the categories. Logic would place the zero on the horizontal line, but it actually appears at the very bottom. This is because the lines are not scales but representations of the relationship between categories. The meeting-point of the lines represents the unlabelled present moment, where the categories meet in the self-awareness of the individual.

This picture may help to clarify the distinction between Berkeley speaking metaphysically and Berkeley speaking as a philosopher. As a metaphysician Berkeley is arguing that the material, finite world of experience is like the horizontal line, suspended between absolute presence ($\infty$) and its inverse (o). He is saying that it is ridiculous to conceive of the horizontal line as producing anything: the source of everything finite is infinite self-awareness relating to non-existence. If therefore we are looking for an ultimate explanation of everything it can only be found in our awareness that everything subsists in absolute presence which is relating to itself through the medium of our choices.

It does not follow that the finite, *ie.* what we experience as 'really' happening, in ourselves, in others, and in the physical world, is of no importance. On the contrary, the present state of everything, including both physical and mental states, can be conceived of as completely bound up with the relationship of the yes/no in each centre of consciousness to the whole external structure of physical events and to the whole internal structure of mental events simultaneously.

Many physical events are superficially independent of the

yes/no choice. This is because they are at the farthest remove from it, and they are mainly formed by the requirements of continuity and of mathematical coherence. These aspects are naturally suited to scientific investigation, and it is to be expected that they will be well suited to mathematical modelling. They form domains which are for practical purposes unaffected by the Choice World within the limited time-span of our lives. The pattern of events in these domains comes close to pure determinism along classical Newtonian lines. But since they ultimately arise out of the set of relationships between inner and outer, there will always come a point where the simple, logical, finite model is no longer adequate.

Berkeley's attack on the idea that objects exist in ultimate reality independently of everything else was soundly based. It made possible a conception of the relationship between inner and outer worlds which was free from Cartesian dualism. At the same time many people label Berkeley as a monist and idealist, and so see his metaphysics as taking sides. If it does this it becomes partial, and his view is invalidated since it no longer comprehends the whole.

When we use words there is always an assumed understanding of the mode and context. Identical sentences can have entirely different and sometimes contradictory meanings according to the way they are understood. A lot of humour is based on this. The pun is the simplest example, where the same word has entirely different meanings according to the way it is heard. There is a beautiful and possibly deliberate example in a painting by Jan Van Eyck which contains the caption *Johannus fuit hic*. This can mean either 'Jan was here' or 'This was Jan'. In the first case it directs us to look at the painting as an external artefact linked with the historical person Jan, and in the second case as a vehicle for the awareness present in the artist Jan when the work was in progress.

To avoid misunderstanding (though people don't always want this) we must be clear whether we are using words in relation to the vertical or the horizontal. Berkeley is talking about the vertical dimension, the absolute, and he is stating in the best way he can a truth which underlies all interactions between human beings. He is talking about the ultimate intellectual framework which provides the context for all our discussions. He seeks to convey a truth which is analogous to mathematical truth: it is a concept of the structure which forms the bedrock of our intercourse.

This truth is even more fundamental than mathematical truth. Where mathematics says '$2 + 2 = 4$', Berkeley says 'there is no other substance, in a strict sense, than spirit'. He is saying that our experience is one interdependent whole, and this is what people know at bottom even though their particular circumstances may make them want to deny it. If we try to deny this at the metaphysical level, in our inmost being, we are turning reality on its head. This is the ultimate objective truth which we have to face every moment of our lives, and we have to seek to recognize it continuously in each changing context.

However there is equally a metaphysics of matter, and it is here that confusion is liable to arise, because the metaphysics of matter (as opposed to information about matter, or experience of matter, or the way we choose to relate to matter) belongs to the vertical dimension. Berkeley draws attention to the oneness and spiritual nature of the whole. The philosopher Hume on the other hand draws attention to the need to face up to the reality of what actually happens, ie. observable experience, and not to succumb to the illusion that it is otherwise than it is. He is equally sound metaphysically, since he is saying that we must treat the finite material world in a way which is appropriate to its status. The metaphysical requirement is that we should treat everything we talk about as belonging to its proper category.

It is when each of them switches from a metaphysical to a philosophical context that misunderstandings begin to arise. Each of the truths — about the vertical and about the horizontal domain — is universally acceptable. The only substance is Being, and 'matter' (both internal and external) consists of observed events which have to be accepted — the hard facts. But when we philosophize using logical arguments we are particular individuals in a particular situation, and what we utter has to be the right thing to utter in that situation. So Berkeley, being a bishop, links his argument in the title page to a particular set of beliefs and practices. He does this as an individual expressing his own verbal commitment, and in so doing enters the human arena of philosophical debate.

Philosophers often discuss what is ultimately real, as if saying this or that could decide the matter. In fact what they are discussing is the way we think about everything. They examine the implications of various presuppositions and viewpoints. In order to do so with clarity each sets up his own standpoint and discusses everything in relation to it. Provided we have a means of translating from one standpoint to another this is not too serious, but a lot of the time seems to be spent on the question 'which is the right standpoint?' Like Plato's question 'who should govern?' which as Karl Popper points out leads to great confusion, this is not a constructive question. 'What are the strengths and weaknesses of this approach in this kind of situation?' is a proper question, but when we restrict ourselves to that our lust for complete generality is thwarted.

It is a matter, as Wittgenstein might say, of the game we are playing. If both sides in a philosophical dispute implicitly recognize the ground rules, they can then play a game which enables them to engage in fruitful controversy, and they can hammer away at each other and derive great benefit and strengthening of their understanding in the process. It is like playing any game hard and fair: the act of submitting to the rules and using all our abilities to overcome our opponent within that constraint makes real achievement possible.

It is common enough today to mock at the Victorian tradition of the sporting gentleman. The mocking arises partly because of the assumption of moral superiority to which the tradition could often give rise, partly because of the lack of self-questioning which can lead to blind sacrifice as in the First World War, and partly out of a sense that there is something very real there which rises above many of today's values. In fact the core of the ideal is as valid as ever: it is the recognition that there is a shared sense of what is fair or proper which is the ultimate source of meaning and worthwhileness. It leads to alertness in making sure that standards are maintained, and that the shared sense of fairness is continually related to present conditions and requirements and mental outlooks.

The need for a modern replacement for this is becoming more pressing as the old formal structures become discredited and fall into disrepair. Many people seem to feel that while major bulwarks like the church, education and the family are shaken but not yet overthrown, there is a constant threat of disintegration hanging over them. The New Right, like Moral Rearmament in the Thirties, makes claims to be trying to restore these values, but these often seem to be based more on ideas of moral superiority than on true personal integrity.

However, political issues are not part of the present discussion. They matter, but they will not be properly resolved without the intellectual foundation of a shared sense of fairness. The phrase does not carry enough weight: we should talk of a common passion for truth. Truth is only found by complete integrity in bringing together what we know, what we don't know, and what we are aware of as the truth poised between them. Many people today would regard that as idealistic and taking the fun out of life, but if so they misunderstand the meaning of integrity. It has nothing to do with moral uprightness in the normal sense of conforming to high moral standards, except that it will generally have this as a by-product. It goes far deeper than that. It means that we work hard at holding together the truth that we know inside us and the world that we find outside us, and that we are prepared to pay the cost of that if and when the crunch comes.

If we make this our aim we shall again and again come to critical points where we have to search honestly within ourselves to find the way. When we have found it our integrity lies in taking it whatever the cost. This applies equally to everyone in whatever situation she finds herself: to the joker, the bookmaker, the prostitute as well as to the artist, mother, writer, lawyer, teacher, priest. Everybody starts from her own unique standpoint, and the only criterion is whether she is true to her own self-critical awareness and is aware that others have their own truth to bring to her. As for 'fun', the idea of enjoyment and satisfaction is not irrelevant, but the word is too light-weight. The deeper we go into things the more we come up against the unexpected, and the more opportunities there are to exercise the imagination in new and satisfying and worthwhile ways.

When Jesus said, 'Be perfect' he meant exactly that, but it does not mean what is normally assumed. It means following our true awareness just where we are, being at the same time open to every idea and every person and every thing, and saying yes to wherever this leads. True awareness for each of us recognizes the meaning of the whole exactly where we are. It does not deny common sense. It *is* common sense, and takes the whole situation into account, including our own and everyone else's awareness, situation and knowledge. Common sense isn't dull: it involves giving our creative faculties the fullest opportunity, because the heart of the truth lies in the imagination.

# 4

---

## GOD AND TOTAL PATTERNS

The use of the word 'God' in today's world presents many problems, of which I wish to concentrate on two. First, the mere use of the word may easily carry the implication that one is in a special relationship through acknowledging the reality of God. Secondly, the word often appears in sentences whose form resembles that of sentences about human beings, and this leads to absurd discussions about God's existence.

The first problem centres round the implicit assumptions of each utterance (used in the wide sense of both speaking and writing). The assumptions which speaker and hearer make when the word 'God' is used have been built up by the whole history of language and ideas. Whenever we utter the word, therefore, we need to be aware of the way in which this history is perceived by our hearers. Among Christians or Jews or Muslims or Hindus we will be sharing our sense of reality with them. To a professed atheist or agnostic, we are throwing down a gauntlet. So though the word is the same, the meanings are as different as in the case of the pun.

So it seems better to avoid it except where there is a common understanding about its use. Some might prefer to use it only in the vocative case. However, some people do want to talk about how they are aware of God and to share the experience, and others want to convey their sense of the widest context for events which they encounter. Provided the way it is being used is understood, there is no problem.

As far as the second problem is concerned, avoiding the use of the word would reduce the waste of words in discussing God's existence. People may as well discuss whether life exists — it is just as obvious and just as meaningless. But the habit persists: people assume that they have a common understanding of what the question 'Does God exist?' actually means. It is a quite extraordinary question if one thinks about it. We give a name to the whole of reality, and then we say 'Does the whole of reality exist?'

Like so much of our Western thought it centres on the idea of individual belief and attempts to intellectualize this. The question grows out of the Western experience, and has been a major preoccupation of Western thinkers. We can accept that it represents a real need which has to be met. However, because of the form of the question we tend to assume that the answer has to be given in pseudo-scientific terms, in some kind of verbal proof that there is a Creator.

A better way of asking what is essentially the same question might be: 'Can I see life as having meaning and worth?' But even that question is framed in too individualistic a way. It is better to widen it so that we recognize it as a common problem. We can then, while still recognizing that we have to seek the answer individually, get away from the individualistic tone of the question. This wider form might be: 'Is it possible for us all to see life as having meaning and worth?'

When we extend the question in this way to everybody two further points arise. First, we can distinguish between three direct answers: a definite yes, a definite no, and a guarded but hopeful yes. The first, we might say, is that of the optimist, and the second that of the pessimist. The third is that of the ideal realist, who is the only one of the three who does not take the answer as already decided. All of these answers express fundamental attitudes to life which are closely related to what people really mean by the original question. Secondly, there is no expanded answer which will satisfy everybody simultaneously. Whatever words we use will come with their own set of distortions. Generalizations will not do. Nevertheless it seems right to use the plural 'us', because awareness of ultimate meaning (*ie.* meaning which stands up on its own without further justification) needs to be shared even though its expression may differ radically from one person to another.

Even in this form the question addresses only half of the question of 'belief'. Belief includes both conception and action. One aspect of belief is the process of gradually perceiving on our mental retina the shape of the whole creation. We reach a conception of the structure of things. The other aspect of belief is the act of committing ourselves in the moment to living out the implications of that conception. Full belief combines both aspects in the moment of decision.

To illustrate the way in which this works we can take the example of our use of sight (via the ocular rather than the mental retina) when driving. Through experience and practice we build a deep insight into the reality behind the image that we perceive with our eyes. So we build into the relationship between our inner selves and the environment a sense of the proper relation between our speed, our position on the road, the Highway Code, the likelihood of something unexpected, the needs of other road users. The list is endless, but at each moment we seek to make sense of the whole situation. The good driver incorporates everything into himself as he goes along.

One of the things that happen automatically is that drivers in both directions develop a sense of the relationship between the car coming towards them and their own car.

There is a continuous (hardly conscious) awareness of the whole situation by all drivers. If something totally unexpected happens, all the experience is crystallized in a moment into an immediate reaction. If we are calm and if our sense of the situation corresponds to the truth we will know and do what is needed in the same instant.

Confidence in driving is a trust that this will happen when necessary. It is built up out of a sense of having always sought to drive in accordance with our sense of the needs of the situation. We must have examined and understood and absorbed the lesson of each mistake if it is not to result in a legacy of error.

Although it goes much deeper, the nature of belief in ultimate meaning has fundamental similarities to this example. Our sense of the reality behind the image of events as we experience them is developed in much more complex ways, through experience, through action and thought and study and meditation and prayer. The interaction with others extends not only to the realm of behaviour but also to the realms of thought and words and pleasure and pain. At the points of decision the relationships between inner and outer which we have built up come together in a single unity, and are laid bare. Once the moment has gone the whole process can appear to have been automatic, and yet in the moment itself everything hangs in the balance.

What is normally called 'belief of God' consists in conceiving that the world is structured in such a way that when each of us responds to our deepest sense of the needs of the whole situation (including our sense of everybody else) the rift between inner and outer appearances is healed in reality. When we do this we experience everything hanging in the balance, and the worth of the moment lies in our deliberately choosing to trust our sense of rightness, whatever the cost. People again and again report the experience in apparently impossible situations of finding resources available which they never dreamt were there, but which are released by a simple act of faith.

I had a striking experience of this kind myself in the computing field, where of all places one would be least likely to expect it. It was a case where a complex program had broken down for three days, and staff were having to work round the clock using hand methods to keep up to date. The only person who knew the program properly was on the other side of the world. I knew a little about it, but there seemed no chance of finding the problem quickly: it looked like a matter of painstaking trial and error. I was aware of approaching it simply as a situation to be faced, and presumably that helped. After an hour or so my attention was caught by an oddity in the appearance of a line of code, simply on formal grounds: there was an 'm' where it looked as if there should be an 'i'. I was sure it needed correction, but could not believe it when the whole program worked. It turned out that the line had been changed shortly before the writer went off, and it caused the program to seize up after a certain date. Even in retrospect it seems impossible that I found it, and I am well aware that it was only because the situation led to an attitude of almost desperate openness that it came about. It was not something anyone could have guaranteed in any way: the odds that it would take several days were superficially enormous.

It is always easy to be distracted from being completely open to the newness of each case. We can easily be hypnotized by fixed ideas of the probabilities. Problems arise as soon as this happens, because we are no longer responding truthfully to the situation as it really is. In this particular situation I was fortunate that the serious state of affairs helped me to attend properly; I was there at the right time, and my experience matched the situation very specifically. But if one were in a state of continual openness this kind of thing would be normal.

Returning to the question of actual language about God, there is no doubt that within a very substantial world of like-minded people there is a commonly understood background against which the language makes a great deal of sense. There are two main areas of concern about people's use of such language. There is an internal aspect — the mistakes in thinking which can arise through partial understanding. There is also an external aspect — the use of language across the boundary between like-minded people and people who are not like-minded. What is needed is a sense of what Chomsky would call the deep structure of common understanding which is recognized by us all (whether like-minded or not).

Logic and mathematics can be regarded as concerned with structures of 'rightness' or self-consistency. There are similar structures for metaphysics, but it is not so easy as in mathematics to detach oneself from the context of utterance. Simply to say that the structure exists can look like a partisan statement, because one is saying it at a particular time and it is heard or read in a particular context. The act of uttering words is itself part of the structure.

The structure I am talking about concerns the way in which the different aspects of our experiences are related to each other within the whole. We can attempt to express this in all kinds of ways, and we can sense that the wholeness is there even if we cannot put it into words. Yet there can in the very nature of things be nothing 'objectively' certain about this: as long as we experience things in time everything hangs in the balance, everything depends totally on finding the truth in this very moment.

We have to hold together the possibility of wholeness and the realization that there is no guarantee of it. The wholeness depends on each individual: this in itself makes it seem impossible to achieve. There is no way of compelling the individual to assent. The only way it can happen is for each to be aware of the meaning of the challenge and the need to accept it. Each of us has to recognize that this is what he wants at the very deepest level, and to say yes willingly to what he is well aware of as the cost involved.

Education as it is normally understood cannot possibly bring this about. It is not a matter of merely knowing facts and 'established' theories. These are necessary preliminaries, but at the deeper levels of learning we begin to realize that the root of every worthwhile study is simply a profound love of the subject which will lead us beyond all existing knowledge.

We get a hint of the nature of true education from master classes — especially those in music. In these, students are taken through the testing process of self-revelation and self-criticism in the presence of the master. He has to bring everything that he has been and learnt to bear on the immediate moment with the pupil, so that he is absolutely sensitive to the pupil's need. Any element of thinking 'I am the great master', however, undermines the whole process. It makes the student into a beggar receiving crumbs instead of a guest at table.

Knowledge and technique and style are an essential part of the process of learning, because they are all elements of the way in which music materializes in the physical world. So a technical mastery of them is basic: it is a condition of creation that every detail matters in its relation to everything else. What the master then seeks is to open out the student's awareness so fully that he becomes alive to the whole of music (including the awareness of other musicians) as a living reality which relates directly to the immediate piece being studied. The way in which this is achieved is through the immediate presence of the master.

Master classes on TV can of course look very much like ego trips. The master has standing with the public because of his status as a virtuoso, and we may get the impression that he is simply revelling in this and showing off his brilliance, and is taking the opportunity to be admired also as a great teacher. That is however simply what we ourselves read into the situation. If he is a real artist he will be living in intense awareness of the needs of the moment, which include both student and audience.

The very greatest artists, such as Rubinstein, become a law unto themselves simply because they have a totally transforming awareness of the gift they have been given, and of the overriding need to share it as fully as possible. The time when this can be confined to a specific sphere such as music is passing now, because the world has lived through the phase of extreme concentration on development of the individual arts. We are moving into a phase where the once separate compartments of life have to be related to each other, because they are all aspects of the one minutely differentiated whole.

When we move into the domain of the whole, however great the emphasis on minute differentiation, there is always a risk of allowing our thinking to collapse. Vital distinctions can become blurred. Generalization is always prone to this kind of error, and I find the tendency in myself. I sense it in the thinking of ecologists, and in the slightly easy optimism apparent in books like Capra's *The Turning Point*, even though there are many valuable ideas present. T.S. Eliot says in *Four Quartets*,

The knowledge imposes a pattern, and falsifies.

The danger is that the pattern will weaken the necessary creative tension.

We use the pattern, however, as a vehicle for interaction and for exchanging viewpoints, and it can change. Eliot continues:

> For the pattern is new in every moment
> And every moment is a new and shocking
> Valuation of all we have been.

There are always creative tensions if people are really awake: either there is tension between alternative patterns, or there is tension between a single pattern and reality. The art lies in sensing how the pattern can be used to open up the imagination by confronting the individual with judgments.

We can look at Marxism as an example of an attempt to provide an all-embracing pattern. It has always seemed to me so patently partial that I have not taken it sufficiently seriously. There are three major aspects whose significance I, with many others, have underrated. The first is that Marxism provides many valuable insights into the nature of necessity as we experience it, particularly economic necessity. Secondly, it provides a mental framework for a third of the world's population. Thirdly, it lays great emphasis on the need for dialectic, so that it is a living process rather than a once-for-all pattern. It is not something which takes the tension out of living: on the contrary, it introduces enormous tensions and gives rise to great waves of feeling and often violence. For all its crudity and partiality it touches something very deep in human nature.

The crudity tends to prevent us from taking it seriously, because of our bourgeois trust in aesthetic values. It needs to be taken very seriously, for the reasons mentioned, and we have to recognize the immense amount of thought and dedication which has gone into its development. It is one of the last of the great attempts to provide human beings with an explicit absolute, one more image to be worshipped. Its strength lies in its offer of hope to those who have none, and in its appeal to the Victorian god of science. This god still remains powerful in the public imagination, even if he is discredited in the eyes of most contemporary scientists.

Like all the other 'total' systems, Marxism's weakness lies in claiming absolute universality. It is the 'all' which it claims to explain, rather than 'a great deal', which is so destructive. This absolute attitude at once raises a barrier impeding interaction with other views. The reason is metaphysical: as soon as we use the word 'all' in an unbounded domain of experience we impose a metaphysical prison on the mind — the prison of what is known to exist or to have happened. This is so false to everyone's experience of the world, where we live at the meeting point of known and unknown, outer and inner, determinism and freedom, that it sets up conflicts which reach global proportions.

This only happens when the doctrine is interpreted in a fundamentalist sense. It is a striking irony that a philosophy which is so avowedly materialistic pays such detailed attention to individuals' beliefs and loyalties. There is the metaphysical self-contradiction, constantly recurring in different guises, that if everything were determined by economic forces the beliefs of citizens would make no difference whatever, and the revolution would come about of its own accord. If Marxism is recognized for what it is, a partial view of reality which affords insights into extensive domains of human experience, it becomes productive and enriching. We come back to the question of where the theory goes with the grain of reality, and the grain we can see depends on where we are standing.

Marxism seeks to ensure that people think 'correctly' even when what they think is supposedly going to make no difference. This is extraordinarily strong implicit evidence for what Marxists really believe — that it is human choice and conviction which ultimately determine what happens. The Inquisition showed a similar concern for people's expressed beliefs, justifying itself by claiming to save people's souls. The idea of saving people's souls by force or threats is similarly self-contradictory.

Both systems are expressions of a totalitarian mentality, and are equally in the wrong for metaphysical reasons. They are based on the idea that there is an all-inclusive explicit truth which must be acknowledged and acted on by everyone. Each person is aware of the truth within himself. The moment he sees that the supposedly all-inclusive truth falls short of his inner truth a situation arises which denies the all-inclusiveness of the truth. Unless the 'all-inclusive' truth provides a way in which it can grow to include the new perception it is no longer all-inclusive.

What greatness our offshore European civilization has achieved springs from the implicit understanding that there must always be this openness to new perceptions of the truth, that the final truth lies in people's common awareness and not in formulations, important though the latter always are. Our weather, our island status, our nautical tradition, our poets, our empirical legal system, our Bible, our best thinkers and teachers have combined to give us a sense that human life floats on the constantly changing sea of experience, and have made us realize that the new must always be expected, faced, absorbed and made part of the whole.

# 5

## PHILOSOPHY

Like all writing, like art and music, philosophy once
written or spoken tends to acquire an independent timeless
status of its own. This is good in that it enables arguments
to be treated on their own merits. However, all philos-
ophizing has its origin in the mind of a particular person at
a particular time. The broader the philosopher the more he
will transcend that particularity and speak to people of any
age, but his particularity will always remain: on a particular
day, in a particular room, he sat down and wrote these
particular words; or on a particular day, in a particular
room or public place, he spoke these words to these
particular people.

Once these events have happened they have become part
of the structure of the past. Once a book is published it
becomes an object which is a mental presence in the minds
of its readers, and their experience of it changes the world
to which it was addressed, and so even the author himself
has to move beyond what is in it.

Philosophy in the wide sense can be seen as the activity
through which a culture attempts to express its overall
conception of itself in objective verbal form (poetry
expresses it in subjective verbal form). It is an exploration
of the conceptions of the mental and physical world which
form the background of human life. Even though it is
carried on by individuals, they are themselves expressions of

their culture, and depend entirely on the language and concepts which have been developed in that culture. In the course of time the complex common conception arising out of this activity becomes the implicitly understood background of people's thinking.

In the introductory talk in Bryan Magee's TV series *Men of Ideas*, Sir Isaiah Berlin remarks (quoting Russell) that the central visions of the great philosophers are essentially simple, and that the bulk of their work is spent in elaborating and in dealing with misconceptions. However, the idea may be simple but there may be no way in which it can be expressed simply and directly: words have to undergo a vast process of living development before they can bear the full weight of simplicity. The root question to ask about a philosopher therefore seems to be neither Sir Karl Popper's question, 'What problem is he trying to solve?', nor the one he criticizes, 'What is he trying to say?', and certainly not 'Is he right?' It is 'What is biting him?', or more politely, 'What is he getting at?' Although he may seek to be as clear and explicit as he can in discussing problems, in the end he is trying to convey an implicit truth which he is aware of as an inner reality. We can assume that he has good grounds for taking his particular approach. We need to find out what they are. Then having to the best of our ability sensed what he is getting at, we can examine and criticize what he says in the light of what his aims seem to be — always being prepared to acknowledge that we may not have understood them fully.

I should like to consider Karl Popper himself in this way. He exhibits a formidable intellect, and is rigorous in giving a detailed account of the basis of all his arguments. Among his many great achievements has been to provide an antidote to positivist ideas and to the superstitious belief in science as a saviour. In his case 'what he is getting at' comes very close to the French philosopher Alain's phrase 'every proof is clearly discredited in my eyes'. His central idea is that the popular idea of scientific knowledge as objectively certain is misconceived, and that a proper view of knowledge sees it as the always provisional fruit of a complete openness to trial and error. The dependability of a theory depends on the severity of the tests we can think up and apply. So our inventiveness is exercised in two complementary ways — thinking of hypotheses, and thinking of tests which will try those hypotheses as stringently as possible.

He describes the crux of the scientific method as 'letting our false theories die in our stead' — a striking modernization of a theological concept. He emphasizes the objective World 3, composed of the products of the human mind, which is 'there' beyond the ability of any single individual to know it all. He demarcates scientific knowledge by the criterion of refutability, and makes a clear distinction between subjective and objective knowledge. He does this without implying as the positivists did that subjective knowledge is worthless: on the contrary he regards it as of the greatest value. He seems to have done for the theory of science something analogous to what Einstein did for the theory of the physical universe, by freeing us from the old absolute conceptions of the truth. Much of what he has said and done has now been absorbed and integrated into scientists' view of themselves.

His political philosophy too, though it is in the main a secondary concern, is thought through in great depth. He is a strong advocate of democracy and at the same time properly sceptical of it — in a BBC discussion with Bryan Magee he remarks, 'Whatever party may win the elections, neither you nor I rule.' Regarding language he says, 'I am bored by discussions about the meanings of words,' and pours scorn on attempts to provide absolute definitions of terms. His strictures on definitions possibly go too far: the process of relating cases to definitions can be very productive. His concern however is with pointless discussions of the 'real' meaning of words: he does not underrate the importance of using language properly. When Bryan Magee suggests, 'Nor have you regarded language itself as all-important,' Popper reacts at once with, 'There is nothing as important as language' (Magee, MBP Pp.97-106).

Most of this I see as enormously valuable, and I think I am sufficiently sympathetic to have a good sense of his central idea. The point at which I begin to question what he says is the idea underlying his thinking that what we are seeking is control. The sort of control that he has in mind still looks like what the popular mind associates with science: manipulative control. He speaks of 'our' task as 'to maximize control over the actual changes that occur in a process of change which is never-ending — and to use that control wisely.' Despite the last part of the sentence, which indicates the essentially personal nature of the task, the words 'maximize control' still carry the overtones of manipulation and possible exploitation. It is a concept deeply embedded in our way of thinking, and it still bears the imprint of the autocratic style of thinking which Popper was so concerned to attack in *The Open Society and its Enemies*.

Popper emphasizes the importance of using the proper method in science: we have to recognize the way in which it actually works. He sees science as justified by results. Consciousness to him is the product of language, and he sees our task as moving history forward, with man as problem-solver and the problem as survival. The tasks in the political field arise from the dual aims of minimizing unhappiness and maximizing freedom.

The broad context of these statements is the general philosophical debate, and in that field they must be assessed not only for their practical value but for the effect that they

have on people's total world-view. We can call this the
metaphysical aspect of the statements. Philosophers need not
only to be true to what they see clearly within themselves,
but also to make sure that its expression as far as possible
tends in the right metaphysical direction. By this I mean
that they should seek to give people a proper orientation in
relation to the nature of worth. There are two levels which
need to be clearly distinguished:

1 The level of the metaphysical view bridging all
   approaches. This is concerned with achieving a
   common understanding of the context within
   which theories at level 2 are discussed, and of
   the way in which they relate to people's attitude
   to the whole.

2 The level of the general philosophical approach
   each of us as an individual chooses to concentrate on, as a result of temperament and
   interests combined with an awareness of the
   current situation. This is rather like a political
   viewpoint.

Level 2 is an area of continuous discussion. There is a
constant struggle, for instance, between Idealism and
Realism, Intuitionism and Behaviourism, and so on. These
are part of the continual debate which is fought out starting
from different assumptions, and part of the game is to treat
the assumptions AS IF they are absolutely true. The debate
forces people to tease out the implications of the assumption
that reality has certain characteristics, and the acted-out
belief is an essential element in bringing the debate face to
face with reality. The outcome often matters deeply to the
individuals involved, because they have strong convictions
about the validity of their view.

Level 1 undergirds Level 2, but it cannot be directly
expressed in the context of philosophical debate, because
any expression would tend to bolster one side or the other.

To talk about the framework of the debate would turn the debate into a shambles: by jumping to a higher level we would short-circuit the whole discussion. Real value is to be found in the disagreements, because it is only through following these through into the far recesses of our minds and experience that we can effectively deepen our relationship to each other and to reality. We have to put our theories to the test, just as Popper insists we do for science: the really valuable work in both fields lies in stringent testing.

Level 1 is where we can assess the effectiveness of the debate and can find a sense of the context which gives it structure and significance. I can talk about Level 1 as long as I do not enter the debate. When playing cricket it is no good starting to argue about the structure of the game. When the game is not in progress you can discuss whether the players were behaving in the spirit of the game, and whether the rules are right. Level 1 can be discussed on the assumption that one is talking in a meta-language such as Popper mentions when discussing the correspondence between statement and fact.

A philosophical idea is tested by trying to see how it helps us to deal with and understand the world: we try to see how closely it matches reality in terms of public knowledge. This is at Level 2. Metaphysical ideas have implications for our individual view of the world: they affect the way we see ourselves, our neighbours and our situations in a profound and subtle way. This is at Level 1. We have to criticize at both levels. Level 1 is more fundamental because it affects the way in which the debate on Level 2 is conducted. An idea at Level 1 can be validly criticized if it tends in a direction which is likely to cause an intelligent reader to misconstrue the nature of the metaphysical situation she is in.

Valid criticism depends on a sense of standards 'above'

oneself and everyone else against which the criticism can be assessed. These standards have to be taken as understood, and it is inherently impossible for them to be stated fully. They belong to Level 1. One can attempt to indicate their nature by means of a set of rules. This is all that can happen explicitly. But all rules are only minimal conditions: the truism that the 'spirit of the game' is much more important always applies. The rules simply point to a common real standard which is external to the players and which becomes part of them in the course of the game. In the light of a standard of this kind, a philosopher can make a criticism which is perceived to be reasonable by someone who shares the same implicit understanding of the whole situation. The standard applies both to the criticism and the way in which it is made: it is objective and subjective at the same time, entirely bound up with the reality of the situation.

Philosophers spend a good deal of their time trying to score points off each other and dismissing each other's activities as irrelevant or meaningless. This must be taken seriously as part of the game at Level 2, but it is disastrous if it is taken to be at Level 1 — as if what is being sought is absolute truth. This can too easily happen, and the risk needs to be recognized. There is obviously great pressure in this direction if people feel they are staking their reputation on some hypothesis or some global view, so that it has to be defended at all costs. That is how Bertrand Russell came close to destroying himself: he thought he saw the 'ultimate truth' within his grasp, and had the mortifying experience of finding it turn to ashes in his hands when he found that the apparent completeness of his formulation of mathematics was undermined by the paradoxes. The frequently stated idea that you mustn't take yourself too seriously is a very serious one: it means that while you must seek to the utmost to do justice to your own view, it is never justified or complete in itself, and the real work is always the job of bringing it into relationship with everyone else so that it helps to open the way to an implicit shared understanding.

A philosophical system is in some ways like a Parliamentary bill. There is a growing sense of an area of need, as many different voices draw attention to it. In politics it finds its focus in a minister and his shadow; in philosophy it finds its focus in a philosopher and his critics. The minister presents a bill; the philosopher presents a theory. There are amendments to the bill; there are criticisms of the theory. If the process works properly, we finish up with something to which everyone has had a fair chance to contribute. This can only happen if it is clear that there has been fairmindedness, not necessarily in the sense that you explicitly acknowledge your opponent's arguments, but in the sense of recognizing a common implicit bar of reality at Level 1 before which all the arguments are judged.

Returning again to Popper, he directs attention in most of his writing mainly to the public domain and to his World 3, the world of ideas, art, institutions, libraries and so on. He elevates these to the status of independently existing artefacts. He emphasizes the need for explicit discussion and criticism, and regards the externalization of theories and artistic visions as part of the necessary discipline required for truly creative work. At the same time he seems to leave out a fundamental element. That element is the individual seen as a centre of choice in the particular real situation.

He is concerned with scientific activity in general and political theories in general — with what is 'correct' scientific method and what are the guiding principles for public policy. It is true that he insists on starting where you are, and he provides the maxims already mentioned, 'Minimize avoidable suffering' and 'Maximize the freedom of individuals to live as they wish.' He would judge these by their success in generating real problems to be solved. But if and when he implies 'these are *always* the questions to ask, in this order,' he usurps the position of the individual in deciding how to approach the situation, and tends to continue the tradition of autocratic didacticism.

His ideas are brilliantly coherent and he expresses them with beautiful clarity. In both scientific and political fields he has had great influence in shaping people's thinking. He is also very subtle in the way in which he appeals implicitly all the time to deep intuitive truths. For instance, when discussing the concept of correspondence to the facts, he says, 'We know what it means for the theory to correspond to the facts even if you can't decide whether it *does* correspond to the facts or not.' It is striking that he is willing to appeal to common experience in making such a fundamental assertion.

However he can also gloss over significant features of a situation. Discussing his general picture of science with Bryan Magee he begins, 'We choose some interesting problem.' It is true that he is not at this juncture directly concerned with the method of choice, on which he expresses views elsewhere. But the function of this opening sentence is to set the stage, and the picture it creates of the context of science contains no hint of pressure or needs imposed on science by the actual situation. It places the subject 'we' in a rather superior position, giving the impression that we survey an array of problems, in a rather detached way and say, 'Ah, that looks interesting, let's work on that one.'

I don't think it is unfair to pick on this. He is a very precise thinker and he is aware of the function of his sentence, and he has prefaced his remarks with an indication that this is a definitive statement. It hints at a slightly aloof attitude. This comes across in Popper's own style in a broadcast discussion with the philosophers Strawson and Warnock (Magee, *Modern British Philosophy*, Chapter 8) — he displays something close to annoyance at having to discuss things which he regards as not worth attention. It is not irrelevant to mention these points because they are part of the message that Popper conveys, whatever his formal ideas and his actual words, and it is this fundamental implicit message which goes deepest into our perceptions of him. There is a convention that ideas and artistic creations are something totally separate from the person. It is a convention which needs to be questioned even in the sphere of philosophy. Like 'do what I say, not what I do', in the final analysis it will not stand up. If his words convey the impression, 'I have looked into the matter, and it's not worth discussing,' he is overlooking the first rule of human behaviour: he is shutting off the possibility of real interaction. Any trace of dismissiveness implies that one is automatically the final arbiter, and this attitude is at odds with the metaphysical truth because it cuts one off from the living moment.

We have already discussed the basic metaphysical truth that each person-moment lies at the intersection of the eternal and the finite dimensions, and that each moment has to be linked properly to the next through a right awareness of the whole situation. This implies that if Popper *really* believes he is automatically right, then he is wrong, because he is denying the reality of the situation that he is in, which involves other people and their opinion. Believing that he is *probably* right is an entirely different matter. It implies an attitude of openness as opposed to an attitude analogous to totalitarianism — as Popper would wish. One basic metaphysical test for any thinker is that he is willing to give up psychological proprietorship of his ideas. This is hard but essential: it is like a parent letting her child out into the world. The idea has to face life, and if it is strong it will flourish.

The *way* anything is presented is a fundamental part of its meaning. It is not a matter of the medium being the message — a striking but rather diffuse notion. The whole message is conveyed by the combination of content and manner. It is through the relationship between these that we sense the metaphysical intent behind it.

Considered from the metaphysical point of view Popper's view seems to leave a central void. It is concerned all the time with the 'real' external world, and leaves us with survival in that world as the problem we are faced with. That is not too bad if it is said in the spirit of 'the show must go on'. But to keep the show going requires more than the right methodology: it requires the vision that it is worthwhile in itself, and each individual needs to share in that vision. From many of his asides it is clear that Popper has a very warm personal sense of the meaningfulness of the whole range of human activity, and he clearly takes immense delight in the tasks that he undertakes. He enables us to share this delight through the beautiful way in which he writes. But in his philosophy he seems to avoid discussing the metaphysical status of the unique act of choice. He takes us a long way towards the meaning of freedom, but does not get as far as establishing a conception of the worth of the whole.

He would probably say that that is not part of his job. He pours scorn on the search for 'the philosopher's stone — some recipe for all our ills', at the same time deploring the 'decline in the rationality of discussion'. He wants to approach the truth via clearly argued rational paths which avoid accepting 'some impressive theory wholesale'. He is right to do so when talking about any explicit theory, because explicit theories, however formulated, remain objects in the world which we have to interpret. On the other hand an intuitive sense of the whole, while it may lead to theories, is itself something quite different. It gathers the whole range of experience and ideas and logic into an integrated and living sense of the present. Just as we can know what 'correspondence to the facts' means, and know that there is some sense in which it can be achieved, so we can know at a deep inner level what 'a sense of the whole' means, and realize that it too is not beyond the bounds of the possible.

# 6

## PARADOXES AND THREENESS

The paradoxes have always exercised a fascination on the minds of philosophers. I think this is because they have sensed that there is something very profound about them. They were devised by the Greek Pre-Socratic philosophers to show that ideas of change are internally inconsistent, and that reality is a timeless whole. Their original purpose, in fact, was metaphysical. It is curious that the efforts of philosophers seem to have been concentrated on trying to get round the paradoxes rather than trying to absorb the profound truth which they illustrate. They seem to have generally been seen as obstructions to rather than windows on the truth.

On the surface they look like trivial word games. But they were catastrophic for two of the greatest mathematical philosophers of the modern age. Both Frege and Russell believed, because of their preconceptions about what could be proved, that their work was nullified by the paradox of the set of all sets which belong to themselves. This shows clearly that the appearance of triviality is a deception.

There are many forms of paradox, but they all centre around a fundamental relationship which can be seen particularly clearly in what is known as Grelling's paradox. Grelling was a mathematician who in 1908 announced the paradox of what he called 'heterological' adjectives. 'Autological' adjectives apply to themselves, and 'heterological' adjectives do not apply to themselves. He pointed to the paradox that we cannot decide whether the adjective 'heterological' is autological or heterological.

To make this a little clearer we can use slightly simpler terminology, replacing 'autological' with 'self-true' and 'heterological' with 'self-false'. Then an adjective is 'self-true' if its meaning applies to itself. For instance the Scottish word 'wee' is a wee word, the word 'English' is an English word, the word 'one' is one word, and so on. An adjective is 'self-false' if its meaning does not apply to itself. 'Long' is not long, 'French' is not French, 'two' is not two words.

Given these definitions, we can prove that it is not possible to split the set of adjectives into two mutually exclusive boxes A and B labelled 'self-true' and 'self-false'. If we try to put the adjective 'self-false' itself into either box A or box B we find there is a contradiction. If we put it into A the fact that it is in A implies that it applies to itself, which conflicts with its own meaning. If we put it into B the fact that it is in B implies that it is not true of itself, but in that case its meaning does apply to itself, since its meaning is 'it is not true of itself', and so it is in the wrong box.

We cannot therefore consistently split this group of adjectives into less than three categories:

| | | |
|---|---|---|
| T | Self-true (which includes the word 'self-true') | Box A |
| 'F' | The word 'self-false' (and any other adjective with the same meaning) | Box C |
| F | Other self-false words | Box B |

The smallest number of boxes which will enable us to handle these adjectives properly is therefore three. We can refer to this result as the Proof of Threeness. It can be put in the more general form:

A self-referent category splits the universe of discourse into three irreducible sets.

If you are interested there is a formal proof in Appendix A.

There is a similar paradox involving statements. We can see the statement, 'What I am saying now is true' as an expression of the implicit understanding underlying all normal communication. There is no conflict between the truth value of the statement and its content. But the negative of this, 'What I am saying now is false', leads to a direct conflict between the implication and the content.

The contradiction lies in the fact that the statement is *uttered* in a context in which both speaker and hearers understand the formal meaning of what is said. It does not exist in a vacuum. Those who hear it can react in all sorts of ways: 'He doesn't mean it', 'He's pulling our legs', 'That's self-contradictory', 'That's rubbish', and so on. But at the root of it all is the fact that the person is choosing to make the statement and is thereby claiming that it represents the truth. He is appealing to the hearer's sense of the integrity linking what is said to what is meant.

The problem looks trivial because there is little point in making either statement: a statement about the statement itself is completely uninformative except about the speaker's relationship to the statement. But there are at least two non-trivial aspects of it. First, there is the remarkable ability we have to stand outside the statement while it is being made. Secondly, there is the strong suggestion that self-authentication is a fundamental feature of truth.

The Self-true Paradox gets close to the heart of the paradoxes. The structure it reveals is common to all the major celebrated paradoxes apart from Zeno's arrow which concerns the relationship between finite and infinite. It arises out of the inherent relationship between two fundamental concepts — SELF-REFERENCE and NEGATION. If these are applied simultaneously both internally and externally they are bound to result in a metaphysical conflict which can only be resolved by human choice.

The idea of reference itself presupposes a human awareness

which applies the reference. The action of applying a category to a thing is a decision made by a person who is aware of what he is doing. Each such decision is a process which links two ways in which we view the world — the conceptual way and the observational way. The conceptual way is our internalized sense of the structure of the world, and the observational way is how the world impinges on our senses. This can be seen by rearranging the pattern above slightly:

| Present | Past/Future | |
|---------|-------------|--|
| T | 'F' | (Conceptual) |
| | F | (Observational) |

We can put this into a still more significant general form by labelling it as follows:

| Present | Past/Future | |
|---------|-------------|--|
| Now | 'Not now' | (Conceptual) |
| | Not now | (Observational) |

The paradox now becomes a paradigm of our metaphysical situation. Our awareness of the present is a self-awareness which combines the conceptual and observational aspects. This corresponds to the way in which 'T' and T coincide. But our sense of what is 'not now' leads to a split. 'Not now' can be sensed as being related to the present either on an internal conceptual basis or on an external physical basis. There is an inherent logical conflict between the two which can only be resolved by human choice. The point of the pattern is that however unified our relationship to the present may be there is an inherent antagonism between the past/future extrapolated from ideas and the past/future extrapolated from external events, and these have to be continuously reconciled through our simultaneous awareness of both.

A simple example which occurs in the computing field is the way in which we store character strings. A character string is a set of characters such as the name of a person or a line of text, of arbitrary length. To store it in a form convenient for retrieval we need to keep a record of both the actual characters and the length. We have a choice of two methods. One is to store the length and the characters separately; the other is to put a special character at the end of the string when we store it. These are two alternative ways in which we can convey what we know in the present to some future point in time. One method relies on the concept of number and the other relies on the physical presence of a particular character. They are equivalent in effect but quite different in their practical implications.

Another way of putting this is to say that necessity demands continual imagination in the process of creation. As each moment comes we have to embrace the internal and external aspects in a new unity. In his BBC series on creativity Peter Evans drew attention to the way in which creative people are able to hold two apparently contradictory ideas together in their minds simultaneously. This recognition of the unity behind what appear to be irreconcilable opposites is a mark of creative imagination.

I called the discussion above a Proof of Threeness. The pattern of three is universal: it is a natural pattern which appears at both the simplest and the most complex levels of our experience. From A-B-C, 'Ready-steady-go', beginning-middle-end, the archetypal form of the story of the Three Bears, through technical patterns such as Live-Neutral-Earth, latitude-longitude-height, nitrogen-phosphate-potash, red-green-blue, to abstract concepts such as Upper class-Middle class-Proletariat, Goodness-Truth-Beauty, Science-Art-Religion we are aware that the basic quality of the number three runs as a major thread through all our experience and our ways of interpreting it.

Threeness is obviously fundamental in the pattern above: the paradox makes it quite clear that we have here a case where the attempt to force the situation into an 'either-or' mould is a futile effort to impose pre-conceived ideas. Threeness is seen in the pattern of research which Karl Popper suggests is the true method of science:

Problem — Hypothesis — Test — (New Problem)

The problem arises out of our present awareness of the situation ('Now'); the hypothesis is an attempt to provide what is missing in our conception of our situation ('Not now'); the test uses actual observation of what we do not initially know (not now) to find whether it corresponds to our hypothesis.

If we look at the pattern the other way round, starting with the situation we are left with in the first pattern, we have:

'F'
F        T

This resembles the Thesis — Antithesis — Synthesis pattern of Hegel. It is a structure of reconciliation.

The idea of threeness gets to the heart of the human situation in a way that is impossible for a dualistic conception of the world. Dualism is directly related to logic. There are certainly many areas of experience where it is necessary to rely entirely on explicit logic. Computers are an obvious instance: the entire operation of computers is built up on the basis of the simple distinction between 0 and 1 ('off' and 'on'). But logic alone is completely meaningless and inert. In order to be of any use it must be related to the situation, and so we must always add the human being in order to complete the picture. Logic talks only about Yes — No. The human pattern is always Yes — No — Choose.

On the widest possible level the pattern can as a link with Christian thought be associated with the theology of the Trinity, which has its counterparts in the thought of other religions and particularly in Hinduism. Many people find the Trinity a difficult concept to understand, but it need not be. It can be interpreted as follows:

The reality underlying life is one self-aware whole.
We experience the ultimate depth of this one reality
in three broadly independent ways, each pair of
which can be interpreted as complementary:

The hard facts of life which are the conditions appropriate to our state (God the Father).

The individual person Jesus who alone lived out to the full the truth of reality (God the Son).

The truth lived out as it is recognized by each person in the community of human beings (God the Holy Ghost).

That is the pattern of one-in-three on the broadest possible scale.

One general characteristic of all the patterns is that there are attributes in respect of which two of the items are the same, while the third is different. This is shown clearly in the geometry of the triangle, where each vertex is a point over against the line joining the other two points. A simple example is father — mother — son. Looking at each pairing in turn, we have:

| Dimension | Same | Different |
|---|---|---|
| Generation | father & mother | son |
| Sex | son & father | mother |
| Flesh | mother & son | father |

This table shows that father and mother are the same in respect of the generation to which they belong; the son belongs to a different generation. Similarly son and father are of the same sex, and so on. This is just one example. There is a vast range of possible ways in which the columns could be filled in — I have simply picked some fairly basic ones.

A further point to notice is that the three items contain three pairs which 'generate' three implied dimensions. This property is unique to the number 3. The original trinity father — mother — child generates a complementary trinity, generation — sex — flesh. Since each of these is fairly arbitrary there is no a priori reason why they should form a 'proper' trinity, but we could attempt to choose them so that they do. It is nearly always a worthwhile exercise to try to structure a particular human situation broadly in this way. You will find a fairly extensive list of trinities in Appendix B which may help to give an idea of the concept.

One of the merits of the Proof of Threeness is that it uses logic itself to reveal the limitations of logic. It shows clearly that if we try to impose a totally logical model upon the world, there always comes a point where the prison built by logic has to concede an opening for the human spirit. This is not self-indulgent romanticism. On the contrary it is a genuine recognition of the truth of our situation. We have to exercise real imagination to find the opening and use it properly. The underlying truth (or meta-truth) of each decision is that the way ahead is *really* there to be found, but it is only found in the finding. We can never tie it up in logic and prove it. In particular any expression of it is not the solution itself but merely an element in the solution. Always, as soon as we think we have got everything completely organized and put into the correct compartments, something arises which can only be resolved by breaking out onto a higher level. We may experience this as the proverbial Murphy's Law, but it is in fact simply a gentle reminder from reality that we cannot get away with deceiving ourselves that it is other than it is.

As was pointed out above, Bertrand Russell experienced this when he thought he had tied up mathematics completely in his astonishing book *Principia Mathematica*. His hopes were destroyed by the paradox mentioned earlier, which is very similar to Grelling's paradox except that it concerns an infinite set. The Proof of Threeness shows that what Russell was attempting was impossible. The paradox can only be resolved by stepping outside the limits within which Russell was trying to work. He tried to do this with his Theory of Types, but this was a rather cumbersome and unsatisfactory device which he himself was not happy with.

The full mathematical proof that Russell's aim was impossible was provided by Gödel in his celebrated theorem in 1931. We might regard Gödel's theorem as a corollary of the Proof of Threeness, but that is a purely intuitive insight: nobody would be happy about that without Gödel's formal proof. Conversely we have to be careful about leaping to metaphysical conclusions as a result of Gödel's proof. Anthony Quinton, writing in the *Fontana Dictionary of Modern Thought* about Gödel's theorem, concludes his article: 'Much more speculative is the inference of the falsity of any theory which takes the mind to be a mechanical, determinate system.' A similar point is made by Van Heijenoort at the end of an article on the theorem in the *Encyclopedia of Philosophy*: '(Gödel's results) should not be rashly called upon to justify the primacy of some act of intuition that would dispense with formalization.'

Gödel's theorem states that in any consistent formal system based on the arithmetic of natural numbers there is always a formula whose validity is indeterminate, *ie.* it is neither provable nor unprovable. The attribute 'provable' is represented by a formula 'P' within the system, which defines a set of formulas P which includes itself. Thus 'provable' is self-referent. The attribute 'unprovable' is represented by another formula, the negative of 'P', which we can call 'Q'. If a formula belongs to the set defined by 'Q' (the set Q), its inclusion in the set means that it is provable that the formula is unprovable. However, since 'Q' is a formula within the system, it can be applied to itself. If this yields the result 'provable', there is a contradiction because 'Q' is the formula 'not P'. If it yields the result 'unprovable', that means that it belongs to Q and therefore that it is provable that it is unprovable. 'Q' can therefore properly belong neither to the set P nor to the set Q, *ie.* it is neither provable nor unprovable.

Escape from the contradiction is very simple: if we go one

step up to a higher level of proof there is no problem. But the theorem is an irrefutable reminder that whenever self-reference is involved it is impossible to remain totally within the system itself. This means that since every system which is created by human beings is judged on criteria similar to provability, no system can be complete in itself.

The theorem centres around a negative statement: it denies that an explicitly formulated theory can be universal. It undermines completely the idea that anyone can expound a theory which is 'the truth'. This is the ultimate achievement of the critical stance — to prove that proof is not possible. The irony is that it took such enormous effort to prove what can be obvious to the simplest human being, and that great minds such as Russell's were the hardest to convince. They had taken for granted that there was a Platonic form which corresponds to the 'whole truth'. The only way in which they could be freed from their illusion was by using the tools of mathematics which had become the only tools they could trust.

Gödel's mathematical case is analogous to Grelling's logical case; just as the question 'Which box does the adjective "Self-false" go into?' has no possible answer within the current logical framework, so we cannot get the result 'provable' or 'unprovable' for the formula Q. We see the same basic pattern as for the self-false paradox. The move from the realm of logic into the realm of real numbers transfers us from the idea of truth to the idea of provability, but the basic elements of self-reference and negation remain.

The same kind of argument extends to computer systems, where it is now well recognized that it is impossible to have a complete theory for an artificial system. Lehmann puts this very clearly and strikingly in an article in the *Encyclopedia of Ignorance* (Page 352). He extends the discussion beyond Gödel's Theorem to point out that 'the correctness of a computer model of a system can never be demonstrated from within itself. That is, the behaviour of the system cannot be predicted absolutely from within the system . . . Ignorance about the total behaviour of artificial systems is intrinsic to their very existence . . . the very activity of proving its model correct is itself part of artificial-system activity. Thus there exists no environment external to the system from which its total and absolute behaviour may be observed. Hence exact system science is not knowable, is meaningless, does not exist.' This is a statement which could well be extended to the whole of our thinking.

The fact that Quinton and Van Heijenoort felt it necessary to issue their warning is an indication of the immaturity which still pervades our thinking. We find that 'this theory is complete' is not true. We then plunge into the despair of 'this theory is useless', from which we recoil into the arms of mystical or political idealism. This displays the kind of 'all-or-nothing' approach characterizing the idealist who worships his ideals rather than the truth. All we have shown is that a theory cannot stand on its own: it must be related to everything else by human judgment. Subject to that condition it may remain of extraordinary value and importance.

The discussion casts new light on the relationship between form and content. At any point in time we may believe we can make sense of our experience up to now by means of a formulation which fits the facts, the content. We take a step into the future, and there are new facts, and so the formulation may be radically undermined at any moment. Even in the most objective and fundamental areas of logic, mathematics and computer models this is true; much more so in all the more personal areas of our lives. It looks obvious, but in fact our propensity for seeking something absolute outside ourselves takes millennia to break down. It is a step in the right direction to have shown that the way out via logic and mathematics has been proved in the terms of these subjects themselves to be firmly barred. If it was not, people would be illegitimately relieved of their responsibility to relate properly to each other.

Lehmann's article has particular relevance to my own experience in computing. I have found Popper's approach highly appropriate. In building computer models we are constantly faced with the problem of making sure that they are doing what we want them to do, and that when a change is made it does not affect anything that is already checked. We cannot do this by relying entirely on some abstract proof that the program is correct. Instead, at the design stage we try to make sure that the structure of the model represents the structure of the real situation as faithfully as can be achieved. We group the components of the structure into natural clusters, and keep local and global features as independent as possible. This helps to ensure that the effect of changes is localized, and that global changes can be effected very simply. In all this one trusts one's judgment and experience. Essentially what we are doing is to bring all-round pressure to bear with as much cross-checking as possible, instead of looking for some spurious guarantee which relieves us of responsibility.

When testing we can use established formal procedures. These can take us part of the way, but in the end the only satisfactory course is to be as ingenious and thorough as possible in thinking up ways of making the program fail. It is no good merely checking that the right results are produced for standard data, and there is no way in which we can prove 'logically' that it is correct. Experience will help us to pick out the weakest points. The critical factor is the quality of the tests we devise. It is the stringency and objectivity and depth with which testing is pursued that determines the reliability of the product, and engenders confidence. While large-scale testing has its place, the number of tests applied can be relatively unimportant: 1000 applications of a weak test may not yield as much information as a single application of a stringent one.

The fields we have been talking about are one-dimensional in the sense that they are areas where an individual studies the inherent properties of logical/mathematical/computational necessity. In the case of the computer one is beginning to move in the direction of the real world, but even so the heart of the matter lies in the formal structure and its properties. The basic mathematical argument is, 'If the essential structure of a set of relationships observed in life is like this, then these further relationships are inevitably true.' If we see two apples we count them and regard them as an example of the relationship 'two'; similarly with another pair of apples. Mathematics enables us to know that (assuming the second pair are distinct from the first) we have seen four apples, without counting them all together in a separate operation. In order to do this and be confident of our conclusion we must be sure that:

— the items observed (pairs of apples) are proper instances of the relationship 'two', and

— the conditions for applying the relationship are satisfied (*ie*. the pairs are distinct and the items are all apples), and

— the mathematical relationship $2 + 2 = 4$ is true.

Threeness appears once again. The first test looks at the individual parts, the second looks at the structure of their interaction, and the third looks at the properties of the concepts which are believed to apply. Even in the 'one-dimensional' case the threeness cannot be avoided.

We can now move outwards from this very restricted and formal area of conceptual thought into the world of human life. The same pattern can be found, but in a much richer and more profound guise. It is recognizable in every field. Broadly speaking the transition requires us to replace concepts and entities with rules and cases.

However carefully rules for human behaviour are worked out, they always represent an attempt to divide actions into the two categories 'OK' and 'not OK' on the basis of an interpretation of the situation. Since they are based on a conceptual model which is an abstraction from reality formulated at a particular point in time, there will sooner or later be cases which cannot be resolved within the system. Just as in the case of logic we had to move to a third box, so in the human case some decisions will have to be made outside the rules. The basic decision is the decision whether the rules are appropriate for the situation. In most cases they will be, but this must never be taken for granted. The judgment must always in the end be based on the uniqueness of the new situation.

As an example we can consider what happens when an insurance company deals with a claim. Claims will be processed at several levels. Rules set out as clearly as possible will be used to decide whether to process the claim at a given level or to refer it to another level or another department. Most cases will fall clearly within the rules. If I am working in such a company, I either deal with it according to the rules I am responsible for applying, or I decide that it should be referred elsewhere. We can call these 'I' cases and 'not I' cases — those which correspond to my conception of myself as I relate to the company's operation, and those which do not.

Sometimes there will be a new case which does not fall within the rules. Its features will not allow me to classify it as 'I' or 'not I', and so it falls into the undecidable category 'not belonging to my current conception of myself'. This entails an inescapable moment of choice which involves my total relationship to the organization, to the world outside, and to our inner world inside. Harry Truman's famous motto 'The buck stops here' expresses what each of us is asked to face up to in moments of decision which are ours alone.

In a well-run company each person will be aware of the overall situation of the company and how he fits into it. He will have the freedom to make his judgments in the light of the situation as he senses it. The choice at every level will be seen as of equal intrinsic importance. In practice, of course, companies have strong external constraints which will impose limitations on the breadth of their vision. This means that an employee will be aware of internal and external pressures which may lead to questions of conscience. There is always a possibility that his awareness of wider criteria will lead him to dissent from the company's aims in particular cases. A really enlightened company will recognize that such differences can arise not only out of bloody-mindedness but equally out of personal integrity. In such cases the proper course is for the company to recognize the difference as a necessary point of growth; if it seeks to suppress the difference it will simply be taking the easy way out and ultimately impoverishing itself.

This provides a simplified picture of what happens continually in society. We build up our ideas of the way in which society should work, and these are expressed in rules about the way in which we should go about our lives. We build up philosophies which help to give us a general sense of what the whole activity is about. The 'claims' in the example above are replaced by 'events'. These face us with the need to decide whether to follow our normal practice, to hand the problem over to those who are better equipped to handle it in depth, or to take the responsibility for discussing, deliberating, and making our own decision.

The abstract structure is common to both company and society. In each case there is an enterprise which consists of concepts, people and things. If the whole is to be in harmony, each individual must be aware of the whole and the way in which he fits into it. For this to happen there must be a sense in each individual of the right way to think and act as each situation comes along. But each situation is new, and there is always the possibility that it lies outside the bounds of what has already been absorbed and formalized. At these critical points the shape of the world is determined — at innumerable apparently trivial points where the individual faces or runs away from his sense of the truth in the unique situation. We experience such choices as hard, but the personal cost is a direct measure of their worth.

The core of the matter is that we should be prepared to test and trust our judgment. Each choice made with this attitude opens the way to fullness and richness in the life of the whole; each false choice leaves a wound which others may have to give their lives to heal. That is what the gospel that Jesus preached is about: to choose what we recognize to be needed is always worth the cost, and each such choice is of equal and absolute worth.

# 7

## DUALITY

Within any threefold pattern there are bound to be dual relationships. The pattern man-woman-child, for instance, contains the obvious dual relationship man-woman. The way in which we view such dual relationships is critical for our attitude to the world. Everything hinges on whether we interpret 'opposites' in terms of dualism or in terms of duality.

Dualism has been a continual problem to Western thought. The origins lie far back in history: it is suggested by the doctrines of Zoroastrianism, and it surfaced strongly in the Christian heresy of Manicheanism. Even Augustine has been accused of dualism in his thinking (by Julian). It reappeared at the beginning of the modern era in Descartes and the thinkers who have followed him.

Dualism holds that there are two independent absolute principles — Good and Evil, or spirit and matter — underlying the whole creation. If we view things like this we come to believe that there is an irreconcilable split in reality. Psychologically there is great danger in this way of thinking, because it allows us to identify people as agents of evil and to put the blame for the state of the world onto them. Intellectually it leads us to imagine that there are irreconcilable problems concerning the relationship between mind and body. Both of these mistakes undermine the building up of a mature and responsible conception of life and our attitude to it. They can have the most serious and damaging effects.

The existence of dual aspects of experience is not in question: they appear everywhere. It is a matter of getting the perspective right. Dualism (with its associated adjective dualistic) is a cruel, limited and false concept of eternal irreconcilability. Duality (adjective dual) is a rich and generous concept which can transform our perception of polar opposites. Everybody has a natural feeling for what it means. A more cumbersome word for it is 'complementarity', a concept which was a constant preoccupation of Niels Bohr, the great physicist. Its core is the idea that each element in a pair requires the other for its fullness. It is closely related to the threefold pattern we were discussing in the last chapter. Proper duality always contains an implicit threeness: there are the two elements together with the linking relationship between them. When we think in dual terms the relationship is not explicit, but we are aware of its presence. Dualism blocks off the existence of the relationship.

As an example of the way in which duality works we can take a general statement about men and women. Rather than concerning ourselves with its validity, I would like to concentrate on the pattern of duality within the whole statement.

> Most men are primarily concerned with logic and
> the physical world; most women are primarily
> concerned with love and the personal world.

The concepts male/female involve a simple yes/no answer to the question whether a particular person at a particular time is correctly described as male. Underlying this simple distinction is the total reality to which the distinction corresponds. Beyond the simple physical differences there are many ways of looking at people in general where the viewpoint appropriate for one sex is complementary to the viewpoint appropriate for the other. The statement provides an example of this: it puts forward the broad generalization that the most natural areas of interest for men are complementary to and quite different from the most natural ones for women.

In this example the simply duality of male and female is linked with pairs which are themselves duals. We can pair off the words in the two parts of the statement as follows:

| Men | Women |
|-----|-------|
| Logic | Love |
| Physical | Personal |

We can look upon logic as the prime dual of love, and the physical world as the prime dual of the personal world. These are very broad statements, but they are not trivial: they contain the idea of a necessary balance between aspects which are superficially different in kind but which are linked in a dual fashion. If you ask yourself 'What is at the farthest remove from Love?' the obvious answer is 'Hate' — the dualistic answer. But if you reflect on this for a moment you realize that hate is the same *kind* of thing as love: it is simply love reversed. A much more profound answer to the question is 'Logic', because it is the aspect whose *quality* is furthest removed from Love: in almost all its aspects it is the antithesis of love. Love and hate can be directly related within the local situation. Love and logic can only be related finally through what actually happens in the whole cosmos: they are metaphysical oil and water.

When we move from one element of a dual pair to another we have the sense that everything is turned upside down. One valuable aspect of seeing things in this way is that whereas dualistic thinking traps us in a simple split which can be hypnotic in its effect, dual thinking leads us from one pair of duals to another and continually widens the perspective. Dualistic thinking concentrates on the simple category sex and on the great divide which it creates, while dual thinking sees sex as a special instance of the way in which the whole cosmos (inner and outer) is expressed in the form of complementary balanced aspects.

A practical down-to-earth example of duality is provided by three-pin plugs and sockets. The important characteristics of the pins on a plug are that they are solid and rigid and extended in space. The dual characteristics of the receptors are that they are (conceptually) hollowed out and grip flexibly and leave room for the pins. So we have a series of pairs of duals:

| Pins | Receptors |
|------|-----------|
| Solid | Hollow |
| Rigid | Flexible |
| Extended | Leaving room |

The technique for making solid and rigid pins is in a complementary and largely independent realm to/from the technique for making hollow and flexible receptors.

The relationship of complementarity always involves a mental switch from one dimension to another. There are dimensions which are obviously natural duals of one another. Perhaps the most fundamental duality is that between one and many, which appears again and again in the dualities between inner and outer experience. But while the main pairings will occur everywhere, any actual situation will call for an act of imagination in deciding what are the relevant dualities in this particular case. There is never a logically correct answer — it is always a matter of what one senses to be worth attending to in the particular circumstances. Duality provides an effective antidote to the habit of thought which expects that there will always be a precise logical connection.

The dual aspects of language run very deep indeed. One of the major dualities is that between concepts and sets. Concepts are normally associated with adjectives (*eg.* the attribute MALE). Sets can be referred to by plural nouns (MEN), and the singular form MAN refers to an individual in the set. Thus the word MAN refers to a phenomenon in the world which we can look at in two essentially dual ways:

A man is a member of the set of MEN

A man has the attribute MALE.

The conventions of language are such that 'that man' implies that the phenomenon we are indicating has the attribute MALE. However the points of view are different: in using the word MAN we are referring to the individual physical presence of the person, while in using the word MALE we are thinking in terms of the quality of maleness. The two are linked by our language, but also have to be linked to each specific case. We find here an instance of one/many: there is a single attribute MALE which applies to each of the many MEN.

We find a further noteworthy duality in ordinary language when we talk about the set of MEN AND WOMEN. When we use this phrase we are looking at this set from the point of view of the actual sets whose names are MEN and WOMEN. We are talking about the combination of these two sets: AND means 'combined with'. If on the other hand we look at it from the point of view of the individual who has one or other of the attributes, a person belongs to the set only if he/she is MALE OR FEMALE. So we can say:

MEN AND WOMEN is a description of the set of

people each of whom is MALE OR FEMALE.

This exhibits the duality between OR and AND.

There is no difficulty in normal conversation when using these terms — we all understand what is being said because we are so used to the way of saying it. Some philosophers have suggested that our language is a very crude instrument because it contains such superficial confusions. In fact this makes it a much more subtle instrument for ordinary purposes, because it enforces a common understanding of the context, and once that understanding is present it becomes unnecessary and burdensome to spell out distinctions explicitly. An insistence that words shall be explicitly unambiguous — so that, for instance, we could be absolutely precise in setting up instructions for a computer — imposes requirements on language which are not necessary for general use. They would be impossibly tiresome for everyday purposes.

In the case above language uses the two words in opposite ways according to the viewpoint. In one case we apply AND to the external sets labelled MEN, WOMEN; in the other case we apply OR to the internal attributes MALE and FEMALE, and we get the same meaning. This is because we perceive the intrinsic dual relationship between OR used for attributes and AND used for sets. When we use language the form of the words normally indicates implicitly which way round we are talking. A slipshod (or skilful!) use of language can of course result in ambiguity.

The dualities occurring in the example can be set out thus (using > < to mean 'can be seen as a dual of'):

| MEN | > < | MALE |
|---|---|---|
| OR | > < | AND |
| WOMEN | > < | FEMALE |

and by dualizing the whole expression we get an expression with the same meaning but in a dual form:

MEN AND WOMEN > < MALE OR FEMALE

The AND in this example performs the function of COMBINING sets. A dual of 'combining' is to select the members who are common to two sets. This is often referred to as the 'intersection'. An example of this is:

The common set of members (the intersection) of
the sets WOMEN and PENSIONERS consists of
those who are FEMALE AND who are OVER 60.

If we use the word IN in the sense of 'intersecting with', we can write the dual equivalence:

WOMEN IN PENSIONERS > < FEMALE AND OVER 60

which describes identical sets. Thus the conjuctions which are used for the different types of operation are as follows:

|  | Attribute | Set |
|---|---|---|
| Combination: | OR | AND |
| Common Part: | AND | IN |

There is an asymmetry arising as follows:

We speak of the people who are MALE OR FEMALE

We speak of the set of MEN AND the set of WOMEN

We speak of the people who are FEMALE AND are OVER 60

We speak of the set of WOMEN IN the set of PENSIONERS

Sets are external while attributes are internal. The two ANDs arise because by convention the idea of AND is used in an external sense for nouns (the set of MEN AND the set of WOMEN) and in an internal sense for adjectives (FEMALE AND OVER 60). The word OR applies only internally, and the idea of IN applies only externally.

In the first example the attributes MALE and FEMALE belong to the same category (sex). There is only one category involved, and so we can regard this as the 'one' case of one/many. In the second example the attributes FEMALE and OVER 60 belong to two different categories Sex and Age, and so this is the 'many'.

NOT is a simple kind of dual operator. NOT FEMALE is (for most purposes) MALE, and NOT INNER is OUTER. When we introduce the negative we find ourselves with a further aspect of duality:

If a person is NOT (a MAN OR a WOMAN) then he/she is (NOT a MAN) AND (NOT a WOMAN) — *ie.* a child.

If a person is NOT (a MAN AND AGED 20-29)
then he/she is (NOT a MAN) OR (NOT AGED
20-29).

Here there is a duality of OR and AND in relation to each
other when NOT is used. These relationships are of course
part of the standard groundwork of logic. The second
example reveals asymmetry again. We can set out the truth
of statements for particular individuals as follows:

| | STATEMENT | |
|---|---|---|
| | 'MAN AGED | 'NOT MAN AGED |
| PERSON | 20-29' | 20-29' |
| MAN AGED 20-29 | TRUE | FALSE |
| MAN AGED 30+ | FALSE | TRUE |
| WOMAN AGED 20-29 | FALSE | TRUE |
| WOMAN AGED 30+ | FALSE | TRUE |

The positive statement is true in only one case, and the
negative in three cases. In a wild moment of fantasy we
might link this with the fact that there is one dimension of
time and three of space, not to mention the one and three of
the Trinity.

I have discussed these primitive logical examples at some
length because they lie at the heart of our use of language,
and are often hidden by it. In the discussion above I have
deliberately avoided the use of the word CLASS, because it
tends to combine the two concepts of attribute and set. It is
generally used in the latter sense, but when we talk about
'members of a class' we generally have at the back of our
minds the attribute which constitutes the feature common to
all members. If we allow this we can regard the sentence

A is a member of class C

to be equivalent to the sentence

the attribute C applies to A

thus allowing the meaning of C to bridge the divide
between the physical set and the attribute. This involves the
fundamental duality inner/outer, which reveals itself in the

relationship between class and member. We can set this out in hybrid dual accounts as follows:

CLASS refers to a characteristic which is judged to apply to an individual in the external world, and there may be any number of individual members belonging to the same class. These individuals are linked conceptually through being judged to have the common characteristic.

MEMBER refers to an individual, who is judged to exhibit the internally conceived characteristic of the class, and there may be any number of classes applying to the same individual. These classes are linked physically through being judged to coexist in one individual.

We can illustrate this situation in the form of a table:

| | Male | Female | 0-9 | 10-19 | 20-29 | 30-39 | 40-49 | 50+ |
|---|---|---|---|---|---|---|---|---|
| Tom | x | | | x | | | | |
| Mary | | x | | | x | | | |
| Jean | | x | | | | | x | |
| Harry | x | | | | | x | | |

The names across the top are the names of mental objects (attributes), and the names down the page are the names of physical individuals to whom the attributes are judged to apply. Again we can make dual statements:

The headings point to internally sensed attributes, each of which is conceived to have its own individual profile externally and its own formal associations internally.

The names point to externally observed individuals, each of whom is conceived to have her own attribute profile internally and her own factual associations externally.

There is an exact duality between the internal world in which the attributes are experienced and the external world in which the people are experienced. Each cross represents a statement about reality, *ie.* it specifies the particular relationship between name and attribute which the individuals embody. One might say that the crosses represent the truth about the relationships in the given context. To establish this truth requires a complex web of human judgments (and records) which link the appropriate attributes to the appropriate people.

The reason for drawing attention to this kind of duality is that it gives an insight into the structure of our existence. We can see ourselves as living at the meeting point of two fundamentally different kinds of entity (attributes and individuals) which can only be related to each other in experience, and not in any theoretical way. The two aspects are radically different: the only thing they have in common is that they are simultaneous aspects of our experience. Because of our ingrained habits of thought we constantly try to link them into a single logical unity, and this gives rise to dualistic thinking. In particular we try to impose on reality the assumption of simple causality.

From the discussion in the previous chapter it should be clear that this is to misconstrue the whole nature of things. In some fields logic carries us a long way, but it is intrinsically impossible even in logic's pure and limited field for it to take us the whole way. To dream of the possibility is idealistic self-deception, and yet innumerable thinkers have fallen into the trap and continue to do so.

Once we recognize that the two aspects represent domains in which we experience real events, and that the real events in the one form the dual of the events in the other, the dualism is replaced by duality. It no longer leads to a metaphysical intellectual problem, because reality is no longer seen as existing in the objects and concepts themselves but in the relationship between them which is established within each individual. It is in the integrity of this relationship that reality lies.

The mathematical concept of a negative can be regarded as a dual of the simplest possible kind. It does not contain the richness of the personal duals, but it does contain the idea of a metaphysical dual in a very profound way. Mathematicians tend to learn to think of negative numbers as a kind of real entity, since they can be represented graphically as going to the left instead of to the right. But the positive whole numbers are the only numbers that we can interpret directly in terms of countable objects, and negative numbers are simply ways of conceiving of absence in relation to the positive numbers. We cannot count the objects which are *not* there. The simplest 'negative' of all is the symbol o (zero), which simply means 'nothing'. The idea of negativity is directly related to the metaphysical concepts of presence and absence.

Among the most basic personal dualities we experience are:

| | | |
|---|---|---|
| male/female | mind/body | lingam/yoni |
| concept/object | class/member | quality/quantity |
| one/many | time/space | inner/outer |
| form/content | individual/community | container/content |
| love/logic | yes/no | and/or |
| noun/verb | adjective/noun | subject/object |
| same/different | rest/change | old/new |
| presence/absence | something/nothing | full/empty |
| theory/practice | idealist/realist | idea/fact |
| life/death | past/future | known/unknown |
| hot/cold | now/then | seek/see |

(The link to the Yin and Yang of Chinese philosophy is obvious). Each pair has its quantitative aspect, as anything we discuss must have, but this has its own dual in the form of the qualitative relationship between instances of the pairs. The pairs do not balance each other in the same dimension, but complement each other in dimensions which are at right angles to / independent of / orthogonal to each other.

It is clear that there is an unlimited number of ways in which duality appears, but while we may seem able to

choose to look at things in any way we like there is nothing
arbitrary about the way in which duality actually operates.
If we work on the fundamental assumption of science —
that the cosmos is a coherent unity — it is clear that there
must always be a precisely judged balance between
complementary aspects. When we make choices we are
always balancing imponderables against each other. There
is no completely rational way of choosing between food and
flowers. One of the main considerations in any decision is
the relationship of known to unknown. The concept of
duality provides a sense of proper balance which helps to
free the imagination. It provides a rationale but not a
slavish method. It leads us to search beyond the areas of
obvious concern in order to develop a more creative insight
into every situation.

In the scientific/mathematical field the symbols 1 and 0
crop up everywhere. They form the basis of all computer
operations. They are linked closely to further pairs:

| | | |
|---|---|---|
| line/point | square/circle | cube/sphere |
| positive/negative | rational/irrational | real/imaginary |
| vertical/horizontal | longitude/latitude | left/right |
| infinite/finite | all/none | class/member |
| input/output | letter/digit | general/particular |
| space/time | problem/solution | wave/particle |

There is a longer list in Appendix B.

At a very deep level we can regard all experiences,
internal and external, as the dual of the pattern of choices.
They are the way in which the reality of the vast array of
individual choices is reflected back to the vast multitude of
individual persons.

It is possible to conceive of this in terms of a structure
which lies at the heart of reality. The pattern of the cross
discussed in Chapter 3 suggests how this can be done. We
can interpret the horizontal line as representing inner and
outer finite worlds, the worlds of internal and external 'real'
events. At right angles to that we have the vertical line

representing the eternal realities of infinite love and logic. At right angles to both we have the pattern of choices which is reflected in the relationships we experience between inner and outer worlds. Each choice occurs at the intersection of eternal and finite, in the timeless moment in which we choose our relationship to our experience as a 'yes' or a 'no'. The three components — infinite /finite /choice — are inseparably woven together in a single perfect unity.

There is a close link between this picture and the operators of logic. The operator BOTH-AND is characteristic of the eternal (vertical) component, EITHER-OR is characteristic of the finite (horizontal) component, and YES/NO corresponds to the component of choice. This is all symbolized in our ordinary lives by our normal walking position. We have to balance left and right continuously as we move, shifting the weight from left to right and back; we have to remain with our head lifted up, as near to the clouds as is compatible with keeping our feet on the ground; and we have to choose whether to go forwards or backwards.

This vast structure of duals points to the fact that complementary aspects of our experience, which one would expect to be totally independent from a conceptual point of view (like space and time), are always in the end interrelated because they are matching aspects of a whole reality.

If we move into the field of mathematics, duality is a well recognized aspect of geometry. The simplest example is the dual relationship between points and lines. Two lines meet in a single point, and two points are joined by a single line. The relationship of meeting is the dual of the relationship of joining. Similarly the angle between two lines is the dual of the length between two points. Extending to the triangle, each vertex can be viewed as the dual of the opposite side: any triangle is partially self-dual, and an equilateral triangle is completely self-dual since the equality of the sides is reflected in the equality of the angles.

In algebra we find a duality between formulae and actual values. For instance the formula for the solution of a quadratic equation provides a relationship between the parameters of the equation and the answer which is true for all possible values. A single relationship covers the whole range of possible instances. The formula defines an infinite set of groups of five values (three parameters and two solutions) which all belong to the set of parameter-solutions for quadratic equations. The groups and the formula are precisely linked by the concept of a quadratic equation.

In computing there is a duality between data and programs. We can draw up a table showing the parts of the data which are processed by each part of the program. The program is a function which links the input and output data. The behaviour of the program is the outcome of the way in which the coding and the data interact.

In the human field, the concept of complementarity is of universal relevance. Many movements today place great emphasis on the way in which we are all equal. The idea of even-handed treatment which underlies this is closely related to the idea of balance underlying duality, but 'equal' tends towards a one-dimensional dualism which is a very poor and limited idea. Women's Lib, for instance, quickly runs into difficulties if it is interpreted too simply and literally. While all discrimination based purely on sex can be justly attacked, it is vital to be aware at the same time of the ways in which the sexes are complementary.

There are clearly many ways in which men and women are interchangeable on a superficial level: there is a vast range of things which can be equally well done by either, both in the home and in the public realm. It is easy to generalize from this and say that in principle everything should be interchangeable. This is to worship the graven image of equality. We have to identify not only the areas where equality is called for, but also those in which each sex has its own unique contribution to make. These areas are of greater ultimate importance than the areas of overlap, because they express the fact that we are in the end absolutely dependent on each other. This dependence in its turn goes back to the ultimate wholeness. One of the areas of difference is obviously that of child-bearing: it is the most clear and unavoidable sphere. There are many other general differences (which can now be established reasonably objectively): men's greater strength, women's sensitivity to personal relationships, and so on.

It is absurd to ignore many obvious aspects of this kind. My wife may not be able to open a jar; I may not be able to remember the name of a person or where I last met her. We each need the help of the other. These are very simple examples. When one comes to a question like the ordination of women, the first thing is to avoid making an automatic judgment. Whichever side one eventually takes there are likely to be both valid and irrelevant arguments on both sides. As an exploratory exercise the question can be expressed in dual form by treating the idea of priesthood as the dual of the idea of motherhood, as follows:

A woman bears a physical child and nurtures her with her body and with what the world provides. Each child has one mother, and the link between mother and child is close and unique.

A priest baptises a spiritual child and feeds her on the spiritual food which comes from Jesus. There are many priests, and each priest points beyond himself to the universal truth.

If we start from a sense of duality we may expect there to be something which is uniquely male, corresponding to the uniquely female gift of child-bearing. We can then ask whether the priesthood is this gift.

However, this is not the only way in which we can seek the balance. We may remember that one of the main dualities is ONE-MANY, and so the fact that Christ was a man may be seen as the complete dual of the child-bearing of women, without any need to extend this to the whole priesthood.

We still have to look into many more aspects which will be critical for our final opinion, but our intellectual perspective has been widened and our sensitivity has been sharpened. The search for complementarity of this sort can awaken the imagination and so broaden the process of getting things into perspective. It echoes the structure of reality.

There are many other important dualities in the personal world. There is the duality of individual and society: neither of these can ignore or override the other without grave damage and impoverishment. There are the dual political systems of capitalism and socialism, which echo the individual/society theme. One major duality is that which led to the dualism of Descartes and of so much of Western Philosophy — the duality between mind and body which is still the subject of endless debate. If we regard the mental and physical worlds as completely independent it is inevitable that we will end up with dualism: there is no way in which the two worlds can be properly connected other than through a sense of their complementarity and of the way it is actually realized in our common life.

This is simply a way of conceiving of things in principle. It is not easy and often not possible to go into great detail. The area of our ignorance is vast, and ignorance itself is part of the equation. A completely logical conception of things has been shown to be impossible. Duality can free the mind from misconceptions, so that we can feel in our being that there is an ultimate coherence at the root of our understanding. If the world is one there must be a perfect duality expressing the ultimate unity of the external and internal worlds. This is like the axiom of the uniformity of nature, which is the fundamental axiom for our analysis of the physical world.

We tend to regard external events as the 'real' events, and to regard what goes on internally as much less real 'objectively' even if it is very real to the individuals concerned. This is a very serious mistake. Life involves a continuous interaction between real external objects and events and equally real and matching internal objects and events. The occurrence of a thought is an internal event which can have extremely real effects — Einstein's idea was as real as the hydrogen bomb in which it resulted. It is ironic that science, which itself arises out of many such internal events, tends to encourage in the popular mind the idea that only scientific events are objectively real.

Each of us dwells in the present moment around which events occur. We experience the situation as a complex of feelings, facts and ideas. We are aware that others experience their situation in a similar way, and through language and all the other means of communication we expand and share this awareness and knowledge. Language allows us to bridge the apparent dualism between internal and external experience: we can have words for both concepts and objects which are linked through the grammar of the language. It also ties us down to a precise recognition of our relationship as unique individuals to other unique individuals, by enforcing the different 'persons' of the verbs we use (first, second, third Singular/Plural). It conveys subtle implications about the way in which we regard each other. Beyond this it actually allows us to talk about the use and structure of language itself — a remarkable self-transcendent property of language which reflects our own self-transcendence.

We seek to make sense of our situation with the aid of a whole array of concepts, memories and attitudes. Each moment beckons us forward to recognize its newness in relation to all our experience up to this point. As awareness of the truth of where we are penetrates our being, we are faced with choices which are directly related to the balance and integrity of the whole. If we shut the door on what we know is the true choice the whole set of dualities relating actual to potential is disturbed: our own conception of reality is separated from the truth, and this is reflected in a corresponding split between the inner world of humanity and the physical world.

Superficially 'just' reward and punishment cannot be expected, because the burden of those who say NO has to be shared by those who say YES. As Job learnt, there cannot be any obvious link between rewards and 'deserts'. The integrity of the whole, the fact that we each bear responsibility for each other, requires that the consequences of any NO shall be distributed throughout the whole structure of inner and outer, taking into account the duality between the individual and others. We can perhaps go a step beyond Job by recognizing that this does not happen in any arbitrary way, in the sense that it is a mystery which we have no hope of understanding. Although we cannot know how it comes about in detail, we can interpret what happens as appropriate in an exact and ultimate sense. The 'right' balance is maintained throughout the whole of our external and internal universe in response to each choice that we make. The reason why we cannot understand it in detail is simply that we and our knowledge form a very small part of the whole.

This provides a sense of the way in which decisions

interact with the present relationship between inner and outer. There are always pairs of elements which are related in a dual fashion. In every situation they can be brought into relationship with each other through the only means by which this is possible — a shared awareness of the form of rightness which is appropriate here and now.

# 8

## EVOLUTION AND METAPHYSICS

Evolution has been one of the most influential concepts in
the world of thought over the century and a third since
Darwin published his on the *Origin of Species*. A recent
example of its continuing influence has been the writing and
broadcasts of Richard Dawkins, whose books *The Blind
Watchmaker* and *The Selfish Gene* have been widely acclaimed.
I propose to discuss his attitude since it represents an
important branch of current thinking.

Dawkins is a passionate advocate of Evolution as the
explanation of our existence. He seems on the face of it to
be the victim of a very simple philosophical confusion, but if
we dismiss his advocacy out of hand we may overlook the
influence which our conception of the way the world works
has on our sense of its meaning. It is easy to say that the
mechanism underlying a process bears no relation to the
meaning or significance of the process. That is largely true.
However, the knowledge that a particular process is going
on is bound to raise associations in our minds. We get the
feeling that if the process is like this the whole truth about
life must be like this too. The concept of evolution can give
rise to the train of thought:

> Evolution is a mechanism which ignores all values
> except survival.
> Evolution has been shown to be the most complete
> theory of our development (so far).

The way in which we have developed is the most
fundamental fact about our lives.
Therefore our lives have no meaning or worth
other than survival.

Because of the hold which science has on our minds, we are
easily taken in by arguments like this. They are in fact
philosophical nonsense. We may find it psychologically
difficult to realize that how a thing works tells us nothing
about what it is for, but philosophically it is obvious.

Even a great physicist such as Stephen Hawking, with all
his intellectual brilliance, tends to perpetuate a similar
confusion in *A Brief History of Time*, hinting that a complete
theory of the (physical) universe would answer the question
why we exist, and 'enable us to know the mind of God'. As
it happens his concept of space and time as a finite surface
with no boundary fits very happily with the view I am
putting forward, but even if the theory was fully unified it
would fail to deal with the metaphysical aspect of the
question.

Dawkins is an unapologetic exponent of a gospel of
atheistic Darwinism, which he preaches with an evangelistic
fervour. He uses TV blatantly to press his own personal
anti-religious viewpoint by means of a supposedly scientific
presentation. The same thing has of course often happened
the other way round, but that does not excuse his
manipulative use of the medium.

In *The Extended Phenotype* he develops Darwinism in terms
of the 'goals' of genes. His summary of his thesis, which he
calls 'a new central theorem of the extended phenotype', is
(Page 248):

> an animal's behaviour tends to maximize the survival of
> the genes 'for' that behaviour, whether or not those genes
> happen to be in the body of the particular animal
> performing the behaviour.

This has a peculiarly self-referent ring to it reminiscent of the theme of Chapter 6, but we can leave that aside. His main new point is that the behaviour of the gene is directed not at the survival of the gene within a particular organism but within whichever organisms will ensure its survival. This leads to the interesting corollary that the behaviour associated with a gene may actually be maladaptive for a particular organism in which it appears.

Despite Dawkins's assertion at the beginning of his book that he is not advocating a theory, this does look suspiciously like a theory (rather than a theorem) which can be tested by scientific investigation in particular organisms. If the theory survives severe testing in a wide range of environments it can become the generally accepted working hypothesis for biology, just as relativity is a generally accepted working hypothesis for astro-physics. In addition Dawkins advocates the main idea of the Extended Phenotype as being of much wider interest as a generator of new ideas and insights, which is certainly true.

That is perfectly acceptable when we are looking at things from the point of view of science. Even the use of loaded words like 'selfish' and 'altruistic' is tolerable within a scientific context provided all the scientists who use the terms are clear about the special use. But there is some excuse for thinking that Dawkins is being unjustifiably mischievous in muddying the distinction between his scientific thinking and his personal beliefs. It may not be intended, but he is failing to be as intellectually honest as his scientific calling would properly require when addressing a mass audience on TV.

Even in his book, though he does point out that the realities of 'manipulation' and 'the arms race' are not as catastrophic or deterministic as the words themselves suggest, he keeps on throwing out remarks (as 'bait'?) which suggest that he really believes the contrary. His choice of terminology reinforces this. There is an insidious use of generalization in the arguments that he uses. His theory appears to imply that the sole purpose of genes is to ensure their own survival. He uses the phrase 'view of life' in one of the quotes below with the hint that it is not merely biological life but the whole of life that he is talking about. So the inference is easily drawn that we are merely the product of genes which use us for their own purposes.

Here are a few examples:

Pages 51-52:

> It might be thought that it did not matter whether the student believed adaptations were produced by natural selection or by God ... My point is that this argument will not do, because what is beneficial to one entity in the hierarchy of life is harmful to another, and creationism gives us no grounds for supposing that one entity's welfare will be preferred to another's ... It really *matters* for whose benefit adaptations are designed.

Here he is so concerned that the student's religious fundamentalism will confuse his scientific thinking that he falls into the very trap that the fundamentalists fall into: he associates the idea of God with a particular scientific theory about the way in which creation takes place. He further confuses the argument by using words such as 'beneficial', 'welfare' and 'designed' (not to mention 'matters'), all of which carry overtones which are irrelevant to the scientific discussion.

Page 56 (after a passage describing 'sexual dirty tricks in insects'):

> This kind of unsentimental, dog eat dog, language would not have come easily to biologists a few years ago, but nowadays *I am glad to say* [my italics] it dominates the textbooks.

The overall message of this remark seems to be that the more shocking and nature-red-in-tooth-and-claw the language the better. It is a strangely sensational attitude to take to scientific exposition, an attitude also found in many TV nature programmes. It is one thing to face the facts, quite another to wallow in a salacious presentation of them. Everything that a biologist says has an air of *double-entendre* about it, because the language has such obvious human connotations and the speaker or writer is well aware of that while pretending to ignore it. Crude anthropomorphism is to be avoided in philosophy and theology, but equally in science.

Page 57:

> Manipulation is, indeed, pivotal to the view of life expounded in this book.

This statement can be defended as simply a statement about a technical biological concept of 'manipulation'. However, the writer is clearly aware of his wider audience. Neither the word 'manipulation' nor the word 'life' appears in the glossary as a technical term. The sentence therefore can easily be seen as another statement of the 'life is ruthless' variety, where 'life' means the whole of life and not merely biological life, and 'manipulation' means using another to serve one's own power-seeking ends.

Page 18:

> [Sir Fred Hoyle is quoted: ' . . . the question that is sometimes asked — can computers think? — is somewhat ironic . . . What on earth do those who ask such a question think they themselves are? Simply computers, but vastly more complicated ones than anything we have yet learned to make']
> Others may disagree with this conclusion, although I suspect that the only alternatives to it are religious ones.

The clear implication here is that if you want to go off on a mystical spree and accept the religious approach you are welcome to, but don't call it rational. And yet Sir Fred Hoyle's sweeping phrase '*Simply computers*' beggars belief as an adequate description of 'What on earth (human beings) think they are'.

Page 181:

> Like God, natural selection is too big a theory to be proved or disproved by word-games. God and natural

selection are, after all, the only two workable theories of
why we exist.

The danger of an approach like Dawkins's is that it confuses
the scientific realm and the realm of belief about the nature
of things. He transforms his enthusiasm about a creative
scientific viewpoint into a crusade for belief in atheistic
Darwinism, and like most crusades it becomes an obsession.

At several points Dawkins mentions the excellent example
of the Necker Cube. This is a two-dimensional drawing of a
cube which can be seen in two complementary ways by
'flipping' mentally from one way of looking to the other.
There are many examples of such ambiguous representations. He applies this analogy to the relationship between
two theories, but it can also be extended to the relationship
between science and religion: both are equally true in their
own way. We can only cope consciously with one viewpoint
at a time, but when we are in one mode we can still 'know'
that the other mode exists and is valid.

The word corresponding to the Necker Cube in the
quotation above is the word 'why?' One mode of answering
this question is to show that there is a pattern which
provides a penetrating picture of the way in which creation
takes place — a picture which takes full account of the
necessities implicit in the physical world. The 'flip' mode
finds an understanding of the wholeness of everything in
personal terms, in terms of an imaginative sense of the
relationships between individuals and groups and things —
including imaginative scientific insight such as Dawkins
displays. If you give these modes the labels 'scientific' and
'religious' for the sake of reference there is no harm in that;
the confusion arises when one side is linked with the concept
'God' and the other is not. We can be aware that both
modes are valid at the same time: one might say that
science gives us a view of the shadowed hinder parts of God,
and religion provides us with dark glasses through which to

turn our eyes towards His blinding light.

It seems that Dawkins regards it as his calling to question the existence of God and thinks that evolution will help him in his cause. This has nothing at all to do with his theories as such or with his status in the scientific world: it is simply a private crusade in which his enthusiasm for his theory spills over into areas which belong to the 'flip' side. He is part of the agnostic tradition which takes a delight in confronting people with 'hard facts' which appear to contradict the concept of a loving God. It is salutary that people should be moved to do this, provided they are simply concerned to attack complacency and not to destroy values. Ironically Dawkins reveals his own awareness of a reality beyond himself: he perceives the expression of belief in God as a self-deception which he has an obligation to destroy in the service of the 'higher' truth of which he is aware. He does not seem to realize that it is this very reality which many people refer to as God. He is right to want to save people from self-deception, but it has nothing directly to do with his scientific theorizing.

He has intense convictions which make him sure of the underlying rightness of what he is saying. This makes him tend to assume that the way he expresses them is right. Dawkins is following the ancient tradition of trying to impose one's own ideas upon people and to expel ideas which appear to be opposed. Centuries of misguided religious thought may seem to give him a kind of spurious justification: those who propound religious beliefs have tended to argue that design in the physical world confirms the existence of the Creator. The result is that the discussion of theories becomes inextricably bound up with religious attitudes. It leads to fruitless and unnecessary confusion.

In one of his hymns George Herbert wrote:

> A man that looks on glass
> On it may stay his eye,
> Or if he pleaseth through it pass,
> And then the heaven espy.

He intended the verse to imply that it was better to see the heaven beyond, but this is not the only possible interpretation. The 'if he pleaseth' says that there is a choice, and that one cannot prejudge what the choice should be. The glass may be important because it lets the light in, or it may be stained glass which is of interest in itself. If we say, 'It is more important to pay attention to the glass' and someone else says, 'It is more important to be aware of the light' we have the seeds of a futile argument.

Whether we look near or far is a matter of individual choice. We pay attention to what we sense to be appropriate at the moment, taking others and ourselves and our situation into account. It is when we force our choice on others that the trouble begins. Whichever choice we make, the fundamental event is an experience of light through glass by a person who is able to respond to light: he has the capacity to experience light and the way in which it is mediated. It is pointless to ask which is real, the light or the glass. Dawkins draws attention to the glass and the detail of its pattern. Theists draw attention to the light. Both are right in their way, but neither will listen to what the other is saying. Dawkins says in effect that the pattern is all that matters and we do not need any light. Theists say that you must simply acknowledge the light and all will be well. The deaf talk to the deaf trying to force their ideas down each other's throats.

It is easy to overlook the truism that what anyone says or

writes is always to be understood in relation to an implicit context. Without the context it loses all its meaning. Academic thought often seems to seek for great over-arching abstract statements which are to be treated as the final word — or the final solution. The significance of the last terrible phrase is not accidental: that horror grew out of attitudes of mind which are at the root of human intolerance and violence. If we insist on the idea 'I have proved that I am right' or 'I have the answer and so I am justified in using any means to implement my ideas' we destroy the fabric of human life.

If we have an idea and express it in a concrete way, it is made public as a finite object. People can then voice their opinion of it. It may be expressed in a moment where everything comes together for the individual. But its expression will at once become analysable, an external artefact which forms part of public reality, and we must move on beyond it immediately if we are to share in the interaction with other people. Every time one produces something which seems complete in itself there is the temptation to rest on what has been achieved. Of course there is a sense in which it may have been well done within a finite context. This is true of all great works of art, which encapsulate the idea of perfection within a finite context in such a way that inner and outer, form and content, are married and become 'one flesh'. In the case of ideas however it is especially difficult to achieve this, because there is such a strong interaction between the expression of the ideas and the context within which they are uttered. Fundamental ideas are bound to transcend the words in which they are expressed and yet the words must be right for the context.

Style is part of the message. There has been a long tradition of scholastic/didactic confrontation. It can resemble a military operation: each side seeks to be efficiently organized and to get its way through superior fire-power, preparedness, thoroughness and determination. When disagreements arise it is a fight to the death. There is a place for a more mature approach. Just as we seem at last to be moving beyond the resolution of political disputes by force, so we can begin to move beyond the imposition of philosophical dogma by sheer mental force. But there is a strong in-built reactionary habit working against this because so much capital has been invested in the old ways.

Each of us is at a unique and equal point through which the reality of the whole seeks to become present in the configuration as it is. We experience our individual consciousnesses as solitary and distinct from everyone else's, and this is necessary so that the unboundedly complex interrelationship of the physical and mental configurations shall be fully respected. Our feelings and opinions and disagreements, about policies or theories or anything else, are the way in which the reality of the whole situation is presented to us for resolution. Authoritarian regimes try to get rid of those who disagree with them by brute physical force, and even when regimes have become sufficiently 'civilized' to avoid the cruder forms of physical violence the same fear of truth carries over into the mental realm. To try to dispose of people who disagree with us by brute mental force (scoffing or ignoring or silencing or shouting them down) is a sophisticated form of the spirit of murder.

It is not enough to pay lip-service to people's right to disagree: the very idea of a right can itself put the relationship onto the wrong footing. We have to digest the fact that if we disagree honestly, that is an essential part of the whole situation, and it represents a challenge to our imagination. We have to be aware of what is happening and of the other person's position and see that simply because he is there he must be taken into account. It is those who can grasp the essence of the whole particular situation, keeping all aspects in proper relation to the entire context, who can open up the way to an imaginative advance which will incorporate and go beyond the immediate conflict to a wholeness embracing everyone.

Broadening out from such partial conceptions as evolution, we can return to Popper and consider what he has to say about metaphysics. Early in his discussion of metaphysics in Chapter 8 of *Conjectures and Refutations* he makes a distinction, with his usual cool clarity and precision, between truth and irrefutability. He points out that any theory may be false and at the same time irrefutable. He illustrates this with the statement 'There exists a pearl which is ten times larger than the next largest pearl', and points out that we can never refute this in the context of the whole physical universe, since we can never be sure we have looked everywhere. Nevertheless we may judge it unlikely to be true.

He distinguishes between three types of theory:

1   Logical and mathematical
2   Empirical and scientific
3   Philosophical and metaphysical

(we can detect the threefold pattern here in the form zero/finite/infinite, or none/some/all). He suggests that the main instrument in trying to determine whether the theories are true or false is critical thought. In cases 1 and 2 this normally takes the form of a procedure which attempts refutation, though as we have seen this may not always be possible. However, in case 3 straightforward refutation is not generally possible. We would expect this, since as we move from 1 to 3 we move from one point of view to the dual point of view, and so the method of establishing truth is likely to change radically.

Theories of Type 3 are not in fact theories in the same way as the first two types, apart from the fact that they are mental conceptions. The first two types provide a basis for facts: mathematics provides facts about the relationships between facts, and science provides knowledge which we are prepared to regard as fact. Metaphysics is concerned with our sense of the significance and interpretation of these facts.

Popper uses his favourite method of reducing everything to a problem. His solution is to direct our attention to the problem situation of the philosophers, and to say that we should use as a criterion for their success the extent to which they solve the problems which they are addressing. Here, however, it is worth drawing attention to the distinction between philosophy and metaphysics (the Level 2 and Level 1 which we discussed in Chapter 5). I agree with Popper that one of the activities of philosophers is solving problems which arise out of our theories and the way in which we express them. But the very idea of solving problems is an inappropriate approach to what metaphysics is fundamentally about.

'Metaphysics' is a daunting word which can easily be misunderstood. It would be useful to have an Anglo-Saxon equivalent of the German *Weltanschauung*, but such heavy-weight terms are not welcomed by our language. The Anglo-Saxon temper is always suspicious of intellectual arrogance. Abstract phrases cut us off from reality when they are used as an escape route from the here and now. Even to mention the word 'world' is liable to make one sound too grandiose, and so 'world-view' is not satisfactory, particularly since it is likely to over-emphasize the external world. Such terms tend to direct attention away from the centre of reality, which is 'always present', in T.S. Eliot's classic phrase. We need to keep closer to the ground, to the reality in which we grow. As an alternative to 'metaphysics'

I would like to refer to our conception of the truth of our situation as our *root sense.*

There is a great deal of confusion between philosophy and root sense. In philosophy we analyse and discuss various concepts which purport to reflect the general structure of things. We have for instance the five basic philosophies listed by Popper which he argues are false — determinism, idealism, and so on: these are discussed in Chapter 9. Great thinkers such as Descartes, Leibniz, Hume, Kant, Schopenhauer, Kierkegaard, Nietsche express their root sense at great length. From their writings philosophers extract principles which seem to form the core of their philosophies, and these principles can be examined critically. Philosophy is concerned with analysis of implications of this kind; problems arising in this area can be solved. They are largely concerned with the implications of logical consistency and the properties of language.

But we run into trouble if we try to answer the question 'Is this philosophy true?' If we try to say yes or no to this we find that the answer cannot be sustained universally: any explicit philosophy will provide a way of looking at things which is relevant to some situations and not to others. The global question is undecidable because either yes or no would imply that reality was closed before we made our decision. We have no prior grounds for saying whether one or another philosophy is relevant to a given situation. The decision rests entirely with us in the moment, and it cannot follow logically from any preformulated philosophy.

Our root sense involves a general sense of the way in which every immediate situation is linked to every other immediate situation. It is a conceptual awareness of the structure of reality. It cannot ever be expressed in a completely coherent explicit form, for the reasons I have indicated. Its expression must rely on people's getting the idea of it, and on their recognizing that it is intellectually coherent in a multi-dimensional way. It proposes that there is an implicit truth which corresponds to the total fact of the present moment, and that each of us has to find his root sense of that and relate it to his own situation and to everyone else's.

A particular philosophy is only part of the whole situation. Root sense is something above and beyond all such views. It cannot possibly be something of one's own, propounded as a great explanatory theory. Explanation is not relevant here. What is relevant is understanding of and insight into the situation we are in, and this goes beyond theories, and beyond optimism and pessimism. For a highly intellectual society it must have intellectual coherence, but it will go far beyond the limitations of our traditional intellectual structures and the tyranny of our 'scientific' ways of thinking. It is something which we can grow into only through openness.

# 9

---

## SOME FUNDAMENTAL ISMS

In the chapter in *Conjectures and Refutations* already mentioned
Popper gives five examples of basic philosophies which he
regards as false. They are:
1. Determinism: the future is fully determined by
   the present.
2. Idealism: the world is my dream.
3. Irrationalism: we have non-rational experiences in which we experience ourselves and
   everything around us as things-in-themselves.
4. Voluntarism: the thing-in-itself is the will.
5. Nihilism: the thing-in-itself is nothingness.

He says that he is an indeterminist, a realist and a
rationalist, that he does not think the idea 'The World is
Will' can help us, and that he can only pity the nihilists.
This is a mixed set of judgments:
1. Determinism is not true.
2. Realism is true.
3. Rationalism is true.
4. Voluntarism is not helpful.
5. Nihilism is pathetic.

I have put them in this form to highlight the fact that
although Popper uses the strong word 'false' for all the
theories, he actually disagrees with them on the grounds of
personal conviction which he is prepared to back up with
critical reasoning. But the main point I want to make lies

deeper: that it is not profitable to discuss root-sense ideas in this way. It is a 'Bang! You're dead' approach which grows out of the whole scholastic tradition of 'right answers': right — tick — one mark; wrong — cross — no marks. And this goes along with the problem approach. Admittedly he goes a very substantial step beyond the old attitudes, at any rate in his scientific thinking, in that he regards solutions as inherently provisional. But he seems always to have at the back of his mind the idea, 'A theory contains implications which must always be valid. If we can find a case in which this is not so, the theory is false.' There is still a remnant of an all-or-nothing attitude. This is unsuited to root-sense ideas, because they can never be fully expressed. We have to study the implications of different explicit approaches in order to get a rounded sense of the truth.

When we talk about root sense we are talking about a sense of the present situation which enables us to relate it to the whole. The present is an indivisible unity. One aspect of it is the process of argument and expressing and analysing ideas. This process involves work on theories: we investigate, discuss, refine and restate them continually. As soon as a theory or a statement of fact has been uttered or written it becomes part of the framework on which the present still has to make judgment. Judging is always in the present: the world as given is simply the presentation of past judgments, and cannot contain the essence of the present judgment. So while many judgments may be forecast correctly, this is never possible in a guaranteed way.

I suggested earlier that the root question to ask about a thinker was not, 'What problem is he trying to solve?', but rather, 'What is he getting at?' There is an underlying message which is conveyed by the total event — the words, the way they are put together, and the situation in which they are written or uttered. The message lies both within and beyond all this. In fact the ultimate message is 'The message lies within and beyond all this'. This recalls a difficulty I had as a child with the idea of the Gospel, because it seemed hard to pin down what the good news was that Jesus was preaching. In the light of what I have just said that difficulty is removed if one sees the good news as the whole of what Jesus did and taught and was. If we try to restrict it to the formal content of his words we are limiting our attention to the explicit part of the message only, and overlooking the part of its meaning which is derived from the whole context at the time it was uttered and lived.

Popper's problem-centred approach is a highly productive one for science — physical, social and political. It has the strength that it focuses our attention on the particular situation we are in. However, there is a danger that putting everything automatically into this form will distort one's judgment of some situations, because it not only leads to clear analysis but it may also lead to intellectualizing. When we intellectualize we say 'this is a true model of the situation, and so the decision is quite clearly determined by the logic of the model'. We abstract from the situation and ignore the most fundamental fact about it, which is that a decision can only be properly made if we are in the right frame of mind. Arguments are only part of the process leading to that. Popper seems to be 'getting at' the need for clarity and the need to get the right perspective on a situation by identifying the problem and keeping all one's thinking orientated in relation to it. That is a very important emphasis, from the philosophical side, but there is also a need for another perspective. This is the point that I in turn am 'getting at'.

The appropriate approach in terms of root sense is to recognize that all philosophical ideas and words, all feelings and all facts are part of the way in which the situation is presented to us. The reality of what happens lies in the depth of awareness which we bring, our state of critical attention and openness in relation to all that is known and unknown. On this view any attempt to express root-sense ideas should be aimed at deepening and clarifying our awareness of the true nature of our situation.

Popper discusses the various philosophies and gives reasons why even though he sees them as irrefutable he nevertheless believes them to be false. He is trying to stop people from going down what he regards as blind alleys. In effect he is saying 'You won't find anything worth while in this direction', and using the weight of his authority to dissuade people. I would prefer to look at the philosophical approaches from the point of view of the aspect of root sense which they are likely to emphasize in the individual. This is what matters most about ideas — the conception of one's situation that they give rise to — and one can criticize them imaginatively from this point of view without ending up in the position of dismissing them out of hand.

## 1. DETERMINISM

Determinism arises out of our experience of the hardness of mechanical and astronomical facts. It conceives of the world as a set of entities which form a causal chain which we can do nothing to alter. This is obviously very close to the truth about astronomical phenomena, and so it is a perfectly acceptable theory there, even though still only approximately true. When elevated to the status of general philosophical doctrine, however, its effect is to cause us to conceive of a world in which no choice or attitude of mind of our own can make any difference to what happens.

This can lead to a fatalistic attitude in the person who believes it is 'true' in an ultimate sense. If we regard it as a global account of the way things are it does in fact run counter to our experience. However, since unrestricted subjectivity tends to regard itself as capable of anything it chooses, determinism performs the salutary task of pointing to realms where this is simply not possible.

## 2. IDEALISM

Idealism stands at the other extreme of the philosophical spectrum. It emphasizes the subjective nature of all experience, and in particular the fact that for experiences to exist (and even more for them to be meaningful) subjectivity must be present in some form. In Popper's advocacy of realism in Chapter 2 of *Objective Knowledge* he quotes Einstein and Churchill as two supporting authorities, and warmly praises the latter's argument for realism as 'the philosophically soundest and most ingenious argument against subjectivist epistemology that I know.' Popper is convinced, and is also impressed by Churchill's remarkable foresight in envisaging automatic observations, which today are commonplace; and the argument is beautifully expressed.

Churchill uses scientific prediction of a black spot on the sun at a particular time as an example establishing realism. But in philosophical terms it is not essentially different from Dr Johnson kicking his stone or Moore pointing to his pencil. The knowledge of the astronomers is much more complex than Dr Johnson's knowledge of the intractable presence of the stone, but both are knowledge of something which we experience as beyond our control. The fact that Churchill's observations may be made 'automatically' is secondary. Nor is the heat of the sun (Churchill's example) something which most idealists would deny. The argument is pure and brilliant rhetoric.

Popper ends up with the dismissive remark, 'Until some philosopher should produce some entirely new argument, I suggest that subjectivism and idealism may in future be ignored.' The phrase 'I suggest' allows him to escape the charge of making a final judgment, but the underlying sense of what he says is that idealism is completely wrong. He may be right to issue his warning at the time when he is speaking, because he may regard idealism as having too much influence, but idealism is a permanent part of the philosophic scene, and rather than dismissing it we should be seeking to integrate it into our whole view.

Earlier Popper speaks in favour of isms in philosophical discussion. What they amount to is a name for a nexus of ideas about reality, and one of their advantages is that once the name is understood one can assume a whole set of implied consequences without having to go through a long list of painstaking arguments each time. Such shorthand labels are widely used in every field of human activity. A parallel in geometry is worth mentioning: if we say we are talking about Euclidean geometry, and if we have a good knowledge of Euclidean geometry, then we can almost immediately derive a whole range of implications, such as that a straight line is the shortest distance between two points. But if we are talking about Riemann geometry, which is of great significance in relativity, a wholly different set of results will apply (and the shortest distance between two points will be what we normally regard as a curve).

There is no harm in Popper's saying, 'For most practical purposes and certainly for scientific purposes Realism is the right philosophy,' just we can regard Euclidean geometry as being the right geometry for most practical purposes. This does not mean, however, that idealism can be completely ignored. If he feels he want to nail his colours to the mast and say, 'I am a realist, and am prepared to take on any idealist,' that is his own decision, and it can lead to healthy discussion. He was undoubtedly justified at the time of his early writing: it was important to take a very strongly objective stance in order to get the philosophy of science onto a much firmer footing.

He lays great stress on his World 3 — the world of accumulated objective knowledge. Important and 'real' as that is, we must never overlook the fact that it is the product of subjective awareness working in an immense array of individual person-moments. If we deny that the position of subjectivity is fundamental — particularly in the exercise of the critical judgment which is so basic to Popper's whole approach — we will distort our whole conception of the way things really are. There are areas where the idealist view throws more light than the realist — the areas of imagination and creativity particularly — and it is unwise to ignore the need always to find a true balance.

Properly understood, isms form a useful shorthand. Just as mathematical symbols and systems make it easier to advance by providing powerful techniques of manipulation and by highlighting areas of ignorance, so isms allow philosophers to make advances by moving directly to the main points of disagreement. It is a technical jargon. But there is often an inherent confusion between terms, and this can outweigh the advantages — or act as a natural defence against outsiders. For instance 'realism' can be used not only in the sense already described, but can also be used in the sense of 'Platonic realism', which affirms the objective reality of ideas.

Associated with isms we have ists. In a given intellectual environment a particular person can become aware of an overwhelming need to propound a particular ism and can perhaps devote his whole life to it. Since any ism is a partial structure which cannot express the wholeness of life, an ist is almost bound to come eventually to a point where it is clear that the ism is irrelevant and possibly quite misleading. That may be extremely painful if he regards his ism as having some kind of ultimate status. If on the other hand he has achieved a mature sense of his position it will simply remind him that there is no possibility of an explicit universal philosophy. The common mistake lies in thinking there is, and it is a besetting temptation of philosophers to fall into the trap.

The need today is not to find the 'right' philosophy, but for us each to recognize the nature of the whole situation. Individual philosophies provide different intellectual models, but they are particular philosophies which particular people express at particular times, and so they themselves are part of the whole experience to which we have to relate. There is no way in which they can be absolutely true. The truth lies in relating them truthfully to each other and to the world, and this is an activity going beyond words and arguments.

Every philosophical discussion is a set of events. These involve objects in the external world (spoken words, letters, publications, books), objects in the internal world (ideas, models, images), and experiences such as intuition, aesthetic sense, excitement, common sense. At the centre lies what I have called root sense (an inner conception of the structure of the whole) which is linked by a sense of reality to the present situation. The root justification a person has for propounding his views is that he 'knows' in an undefinable but real sense that they are what is called for from him at the time they are expressed.

It may seem that I am denying the possibility of objectivity in favour of subjectivity, thus appearing to be a idealist and not a realist. That would be a mistaken conclusion. What I am trying to convey is that true awareness implies and true realism requires the union of subjective and objective, in the normal sense of inner private experience and outer public experience. There is no arbitrariness about it. There is no ignoring or flouting of ordinary ethical standards, nor any blind adherence to them. True subjectivity recognizes and responds to the objective truth.

Nor is this a kind of transcendental monism. Every person-moment occurs within a given context. Even the process of abstract thinking is subject to this condition: it occurs when the person is in particular circumstances, and the thought itself takes a particular form. T.S. Eliot talks about 'the passage which we did not take', and we easily imagine that this has some sort of reality, but the only reality it has is what happens in our minds when we conceive of the possibility.

As each moment passes a vast multitude of decisions is made, which in turn establish the conditions of the moment which follows. We can conceive of each person-moment as having the potential of complete fulfilment within its particular constraints, and can think of choosing that as the 'right' decision at that point. It is clear that this gives us a notional criterion for perfect action, which is partially related to, but never wholly defined by, what we normally think of as 'ideals'. This is what the injunction 'be perfect' means: not an impossible ideal, but simply a full involvement of one's being in the needs of the present situation, sharing a common implicit root sense with others. Since the 'right' decision is related to the whole, it is in some sense dependent on the decisions made by others, as well as on many other unknown factors. So it is always an act of faith — not of blind faith, because one of the normal requirements is that one should be as informed as one can be, but of faith which senses the point at which the need for decision overrides the need to search further for preparatory knowledge.

If we act 'in good faith' our decisions can work together not despite but because of the fact that they are free and independent. They can work together if each of us seeks truly to be aware of the needs of the present at the proper level. That level is beyond the level of 'You ought to do this' or 'You must never do that'. It is the level at which the individual senses what is right, taking everyone and everything of which she is conscious into account, as a matter of direct awareness.

Summing up, there cannot possibly be a single explicit philosophy which is universally valid. To think in terms of such a philosophy is an anachronistic legacy of the tradition of the primacy of the intellect and of authoritarian conceptions of knowledge. Certainly philosophies are an invaluable discipline for developing intellectual sensitiveness, but unless the lesson has been learnt that there is no right answer except the unpredictable but responsible 'right answer' here and now, the sensitiveness is misplaced.

There is in people's ordinary language a particularly sensitive and discriminating indicator of their frame of mind. The difference between 'all' and 'most', or between 'all' and 'some', is crucial. It reflects the difference between infinite and finite. The lesson has been hammered home in history time and time again and is still blindly ignored by those of fundamentalist mentality. If A knows *all* the truth he can claim power over B. If A knows *most* of the truth in quantitative terms B can still know a portion of the truth which can be qualitatively balanced against A's. To claim to know *all* of the truth is a hidden bid for absolute power and is in the end self-defeating because it overrides the truth of the other person. To claim to know *some* of the truth is simply to seek to contribute to the common good.

Having digressed somewhat we can now return to the remaining isms on Popper's list.

## 3. IRRATIONALISM

The third philosophy is irrationalism, which appears to be directly opposed to Popper's rationalism. Once again it is a question of the context in which we are talking. If we are talking universally both rationalism and irrationalism are incomplete but complementary. If we ask what irrationalism is getting at, one answer is that it emphasizes that a very fundamental part of our experience is our immediate apprehension of things-in-themselves, as opposed to our analysis of them.

Among such experiences is Popper's immediate apprehension of irrationalism as a thing-in-itself. This immediate apprehension includes his awareness of all the errors to which the doctrine can give rise, as well as his memories of all the people who have been advocates of the doctrine. It leads him to attack irrationalism. But there remains the familiar paradox that his attack arises out of his irrational — or (less pejoratively) non-rational — apprehension. The exercise of reason is itself a non-rational activitty.

His outright attack on irrationalism seems an unnecessary attempt to impose rationalism. Like realism, rationalism is a highly desirable general philosophy for the scientific domain and for much of the public domain, but it is not universally appropriate. It is what is normally entailed by an honest sense of responsibility in those domains, but it derives its validity from that fact and not from the supposed fact that it is right and irrationalism is wrong.

Rationalism has been espoused by many of the most morally sensitive minds over the last few centuries, though even it has its cranky exponents, especially among the anti-religious. It calls for a high level of integrity and a willingness to follow where the facts lead. These qualities are admirable, and have led to enlightened thinking in many fields. But because so much of the work has been an uphill battle against traditional religion, rationalism can be blind to the fact that there may be a baby in the religious/irrationalist view which it carelessly throws out with the bath-water.

With regard to the concept of the 'thing-in-itself', this was used by many German philosophers including Kant. It is inherently unsatisfactory because a 'thing' is normally associated with non-personal objects, and they were actually trying to talk about the reality beyond both objects and persons. Formal philosophy limits itself as much as possible to what can be formally and explicitly expressed, but continually reaches stages where it has to point beyond. When it does so it is better to avoid phrases which diminish the significance of what they denote.

## 4. VOLUNTARISM

Popper hardly discusses Voluntarism: he simply says that he is sure it cannot help us to possess 'anything like full knowledge of the real world with its infinite richness and beauty.'

Voluntarism is linked especially with Schopenhauer. In his book on Schopenhauer (P.141) Bryan Magee describes Schopenhauer's use of the word 'Will' for being-in-itself as 'nothing short of an intellectual catastrophe'. Schopenhauer's intention is that we should understand by 'Will' the genus which has our own will as its most important species, and he expects us to form the necessary extrapolation of the concept. Accordingly many of the particular associations of the word 'Will' are misleading. What he seems to be talking about is close to the idea of presence. This term seems preferable because it can be associated with people, things or places and their interrelationships. It carries the overtones of worth and *gravitas* when used in the sense of the presence of a distinguished man or woman. The title of his book, *The World as Will and Representation*, might usefully be amended to *The World as Presence and Relationship*, the subtitle of the present book. This phrase forms a fair summary of my own view, and it may also be close to the truth which Schopenhauer had in mind.

The idea of will as central contains a kernel of truth, and so it is not good to reject voluntarism out of hand. It conveys the sense that intention and decision lie very close to the heart of our relation to each other and to the universe. But it is no help to present it in the stark form in which it is often portrayed, as sheer will-power. It is no help to talk as Schopenhauer does in terms of 'an underlying drive which ultimately is undifferentiated' (Magee, P.139). This carries such strong overtones of blind force as to be totally misleading, whatever the apparent gain in philosophical unification. Schopenhauer seems to have been misled by his own use of the term into an outright pessimism which derives from just such a misconception. The centre of choice lies deep, but it is anything but a blind drive: it is the seat of integrity relating inner to outer with great precision.

Voluntarism is open to criticism on these grounds, but it also draws attention to the creativity within each of us which can contribute to the transfiguration of everything. This is no illusion but a plain statement of fact. We can choose to allow this creativity to be freed by maintaining a deliberate hidden and sustained assent to the opportunities that open up.

### 5. NIHILISM
It is not enough to pour scorn or pity on those who are really convinced that the thing-in-itself is nothingness. They are the people who are bearing the burden of our misconceptions of reality, and who are deprived of all sense of meaning. In accepting this vacuum into themselves, and in transmuting it into art and philosophy, they are working at the frontiers of the struggle to transfigure sheer necessity. They cry from the depths, and as long as it is a genuine cry we have to listen with respect, contrition and awe. As long as it is needed to draw attention to the critical nature of the situation the cry must be taken seriously.

Popper's criticism may be justified if nihilism or existentialism turns into a self-indulgent excuse for wallowing in a mire of indolence and self-pity. A philosophy tending in this direction is suspect from the start. But if it leads to an awareness of the nakedness of the soul in facing the apparently overwhelming odds of existence, it is a salutary reminder of the magnitude of the task and the need for each of us to bring every resource we can to bear on it.

Popper respects and understands writers such as Hume and Berkeley who put forward the ideas he criticizes, but his authoritative dismissal of views which they defend may make people think that there is nothing of major value in them. That is perhaps the main criticism to be made of his comments. Popper himself warns against trying to be too precise or dogmatic, or giving final answers. He turned his back on the excessive dogmatism of the Logical Positivists. Yet he is strongly affected by their passion for cutting out the diffuseness of speculative thought and getting down to hard fact.

So he always speaks in clear and precise terms. This is wholly beneficial in his discussion of science: it cuts out the rubbish and gets quickly to the core of the matter. He then goes on to talk about the truth or otherwise of philosophical theories, and here he continues to use a category which has an inherent either/or quality about it. The category of truth in this narrow sense is simply not relevant to the richness of a carefully worked out philosophy. Popper claims to be a realist, but if you take that to its logical conclusion you leave no room for the imagination. Any philosophical principle raised to absolute status will become a false image. What one is interested in is the illuminating insights and the practical implications of a philosophy, and the way in which it conflicts with or is complementary to other viewpoints. As a philosopher of science Popper may be largely justified in dismissing the philosophies we have discussed. When he condemns them in a wider context as he seems to do he is limiting himself in much the same way as the Vienna Circle limited themselves by their Positivist assumptions.

In general, philosophic systems assume a certain environment for their arguments, and since this is always limited in some way they can never be universally valid. The one thing that is universally valid is the need to move in the direction of wholeness within each situation. For any defined external situation this can take diametrically opposite forms according to the real internal states at the time.

# 10

## THE PERSON OF CHRIST

Having set out a viewpoint on philosophy, I should like to move to a realm which is closely related but very distinct, that of religion. The history of the two is closely interwoven, and the same is true in my own history. Much of the thinking which forms the basis of my philosophical views has its origins in the religious realm, and it would be wrong to conceal this. On the other hand if the religious side was the origin, the form of my thinking has been very much shaped by rational criticism. In the preceding chapters I have been wearing a metaphysical hat, trying to discuss the whole human situation as a structure and to point out some of the main features of that structure. In the light of the concept of duality, however, it seems right that I should give the reader some idea of the dual side of the general viewpoint that I have been describing and should indicate something of the personal background.

The core of it lies in the experience mentioned in the preface. It occurred in the context of the Christian religion, but while it was linked to the person of Christ himself and partly shaped by Christian thinking, it went well beyond the formal limits of Christianity. It recognized Christ as transcending all particular religions including that which takes its name from him. While many prophets, poets and thinkers have revealed different aspects of the truth, there has been no one who has lived out the whole truth in such integrated fullness.

While questioning the idea of a necessary connection with historic Christianity, I have to acknowledge how much Christian thinking (when it has been truly universal) has contributed to my background. It is hard to know how much of my thinking and language springs out of the Anglican tradition of scholarship which is so interwoven with English history. The peculiar position of the Established Church, while it has many unsatisfactory effects, has meant that it has constantly had to grapple with the practical problems of relating to the whole life of the country. The universality and comprehensiveness of its outlook has at its best nurtured an attitude of generosity and tolerance.

My roots are in Northumbria, where many of the foundations of Western civilization were laid in the seventh century by the monks of Lindisfarne and Jarrow. Bede's writings and thinking are strikingly modern in their approach, and the era stands out as a brilliant period of intellectual and artistic creativity. The monks still seem to be a palpable presence in the area. The line back through the Irish saints brought an open and independent spirit which acted as a fertilizing complement to Augustine's Roman church. The meeting of the two streams resulted in the union at the Synod of Whitby which avoided divisive conflict and provided a model of reconciliation which has lingered in the national memory.

Born and christened in Chester-le-Street, where the bones of Cuthbert lay for over a century long before the Conquest, and spending my teens in Durham, I experienced this as very much part of my environment. The problems I was concerned about were on the surface Christian problems, and the most fundamental one was the problem of evil. It was the clarification of the nature of this problem which was for me the most immediately significant aspect of what happened.

There is no need to go into the details of the experience. It arose out of an intense period of study. It was destructive of normal life on one level, and highly integrating on another. I felt the need to share it and took action to do so which went outside the bounds of convention.

Although I realized that it would be hard to translate the simplicity of the perception into language, there was an undeniable objectivity and wholeness about it. My critical faculties were satisfied beyond anything I had imagined possible.

There was a cascade of images and thoughts. The verbal forms which came immediately to mind were very simple, centring around the duality between Love and mathematics (by mathematics I meant the structures of logical constraint which I would now prefer to associate with the concept of form). The metaphysical picture was that our relationship to and through space-time is being filled out by Love subject to the constraints imposed by Love on itself. These self-imposed constraints include willingness to allow each person-moment, in which awareness has the direct experience of seeming to be separated from itself, to choose between rejecting and participating in the act of creation.

It was at once obvious that this removed the problem of evil from the metaphysical realm (where it had always seemed to present an intractable intellectual obstacle to a cooherent view of the structure of things) to the realm of actual living. To say that the problem of evil is solved does not help, because the offence of evil is always a real experience and to talk in terms of a solution as if to a mathematical problem would be quite wrong. But one can say that the formal metaphysical problem of evil is illusory. Life is not an everlasting battle between absolute good and absolute evil, but an activity of self-discovery in which we are confronted with absolute choices. Love seeks without compulsion to fill out and transform the whole, while allowing negative choices to have their necessary effect.

One of the images which recurred was that of the Cross. It seemed to exhibit a precise match of content and form. It was the physical means by which Christ was crucified, and at the same time its shape suggests the core of his message. It is simultaneously the shape of a man with arms outstretched, and the abstract shape of our metaphysical situation. It symbolizes the four points of the compass; it also symbolizes heaven and earth with the finite inner and outer worlds suspended in balance. What is ultimately significant — our choice — lies at the point where these dimensions meet in a human being.

Two texts from St John's Gospel were particularly relevant. The first (16:13) was: 'When he, the Spirit of Truth, is come, he will guide you into all truth', and the second (16:25): 'The time cometh when I . . . shall shew you plainly of the Father'. These seemed to say that the message of Christ was about an immediate perception of the reality of our situation, wherever we are. Religion and religious language are valuable just so far as they bring us to the point where they themselves are part of our immediate awareness of reality.

There is no doubt that religions have been a vehicle for many essential components of the truth. Our general insight into the human condition as a whole has its roots in the acts of faith of innumerable people of all kinds. These have built up a vast reservoir of spiritual realism. This insight is true religion, which arises out of a profound respect for the truth which we find within and between ourselves. Particular religions, however, are unavoidably partial: they arise in particular groups within humanity and translate the whole truth into the forms which are appropriate for those groups. The universal truth made plain in Christ goes beyond the conception of any particular religion, and transcends any limitations we try to impose on it.

Two immediate problems arose. The first was that though I could see myself that this made possible a consistent view of our whole existence, it was only a subjective view and there was no way in which it could be proved to be true. The second was that the centrality of Christ appeared on the surface to imply that Christianity was the true religion. This has always led to the anomaly of seeking converts to a particular body rather than pointing to the truth. It is a barrier against communication with those of a different faith or none at all.

The first problem arises out of the mistaken idea that proof is possible. Many people have attacked this in this century, and the point has already been discussed. We are talking about truth at the meeting-place of everything subjective and objective. This calls for an immediate awareness which recognizes that its expression must always be open to question, and can never be 'proved'. We each have to come to an awareness of the same inner truth in our own special way, and questioning is an essential part of finding that way. It is through openness to questioning that we consolidate the truth of what is initially subjective.

The second problem arises out of the hidden assumption that Christianity has some sort of copyright on Christ. Simply to state it in that way is to reveal the absurdity of the idea. One of the texts often quoted in support is: 'No man comes to the Father but by me' (John 14:6). But this is to be interpreted as referring to the whole reality of what Christ is, and not merely the partial representation of his reality available through the Church. One can go as far as to see the Muslim civilization as a kind of first-fruits of Christ's presence, in some ways closer to what he was about than formal Christian civilization. There are new elements in it, a freshness of outlook and a great sensitivity which are expressed particularly strikingly in the beauty and flow of the writing and architecture; also in the pioneering scholarship in science, history and philosophy. One feels instinctively that these are a manifestation of the spirit of Christ.

So despite the Christian background there is no specifically Christian aspect of the perception apart from the centrality of Christ, which is a universal thing. The whole idea of claiming superiority because of one's special relationship to Christ, as the Christian Church is always tempted to do, is self-defeating and stands condemned by Christ himself. It is an attempt to sit in the place of honour. The centrality of Christ does not lie in the claim that he is the 'Son of God' except insofar as that is an attempt to put into words the essential reality of what he is. Any form of words can only be understood in the light of a commonly assumed context, and this particular form of words becomes less helpful as time goes on.

Our thinking about Christ is confused. It is overgrown with the accretions of centuries in which the inheritors of the ancient authoritarian ideas have striven to incorporate him into their structures. We have lost the sense of astonishing freshness which the crowds around him must have experienced at first hand. Scientific categories become secondary in the neighbourhood of such a person: space and time themselves are transfigured. We get some sense of this in the presence of any great leader. In the presence of Christ people clearly met a transforming quality which lifted each moment to a level of absolute completeness within its own terms. To describe what 'really' happened in these circumstances we are dependent on what people experienced, and this is in the nature of things impossible to pin down precisely: we have to make our own judgment.

Christ's life was real: he took into himself the unresolved conflicts between inner and outer states as they were presented to him in their particularity. He taught the simple truth which was waiting for recognition within the great traditions of the Jews. He faced the suffering and ignorance around him and transfigured them through the sheer power of imaginative love, acceptance and openness. As he met particular cases of need he allowed wholeness to fill the local situation.

There are no rational grounds for dismissing out of hand something which on the face of it looks as unlikely as the feeding of the five thousand. We can say that we find such reports impossible to believe or imagine. That is understandable with our mental background, but it has no other justification than that what is reported appears to disregard the normal 'laws of nature' and sounds like a conjuring trick. It may be difficult to imagine, but it is not conceptually untenable, and it does not bear the stamp of a trick. It can be a true account of what people experience when presence transforms the space around them to a depth which goes beyond our 'normal' experience. It can be seen as arising out of the seamlessness of Christ's life, and as what happens naturally in the neighbourhood of such depth of presence.

Christ's centrality lies in the sheer fact of his openness to each moment. He was continually in the same eternal position as each of us. He lived his life at the meeting point of knowing and not knowing, experiencing and taking into himself the conflict between appearance and reality, and accepting the cost involved. But there is no point in arguing this case: there is no way in which I can or wish to prove it. It seems to me an immediate apprehension which makes sense of where we are now. I am aware of his presence as penetrating to the deepest level of our existence in a way which is necessary and sufficient to transfigure our whole internal and external state.

The difference between him and us is a matter of completeness. Throughout his life he is aware who and where he is, and he allows reality to penetrate to the heart of each situation. He experiences the sense of powerlessness which we all experience at times, in the most extreme and apparently most unjust form. This involves the appallingly sudden transition from a successful and happy life as a healer and teacher, and his ecstatic welcome by the people into Jerusalem, to a degrading death at the hands of the establishment. He enters fully into this shattering experience. While sharing in the desolation of everyone who feels forsaken by love, with the terrible cry 'Why have you forsaken me?', he at once transfigures it with simple trust that the experience is necessary, and that love is present at the heart of it. It is hard to deny that for a person who is so fully aware of the truth to live through its apparently utter negation is to leave an indelible signature on the metaphysical fabric of the world.

To end this chapter on my own religious viewpoint, it seems worth giving a contemporary version of the Creation story. Scientists are concerned to trace exactly what 'happened' in the first few moments of the Big Bang, and some of them imagine that that will give them an insight into the nature of God and perhaps establish whether he exists. That is a simple intellectual mistake made by those who should know better. Beginnings and ends belong to the dimension of finiteness and so have no ultimate reality in themselves. Any creation theory simply gives an AS IF answer to how we conceive of the beginnings of the universe in time. Time itself is an aspect of creation.

We get nearer the truth if we say that the really significant 'Big Bang' occurred when Eve took the apple and Adam connived. This truth underlies many different myths. However, the form of the myths can give rise to misunderstandings outside the culture within which they have grown up. Since many 'modern' people no longer like the simple pictorial imagery of the Genesis story, even though it portrays the essential truth with beautiful simplicity, I will try to put it in abstract terms. We perhaps need a version which shows a proper respect for the requirements of science.

We can start with the idea that the need is for creation to come about through free agents. It is conceivable that each person would respond truly to his own awareness of each situation, so that inner and outer were continuously married. For this to happen everyone would have to say 'yes' all the time to his recognition of reality. There would in that situation be a clear run for humanity, integrating and transfiguring the complexity of their interrelationships in one continuous act of creation. This was a theoretical possibility, conceivable but difficult for us to imagine. It would depend on everyone choosing rightly at every moment. We would assess its probability as zero, and we might humanly say that there would be no point in setting up a universe on that basis.

Alternatively there could be a mixture of yeses and noes. Some would say no to what they knew within themselves because they allowed themselves to be deceived by appearances. This is the way it has in fact turned out, and the structure of our universe is a reflection of this fact. The way in which the process of creation is presented to us has to respect this. We have a world in which people have experienced their own and others' denial of the truth. One might say that we have a world which has lost its nerve. The relation between external conditions and people's internal states corresponds exactly to the yeses and noes.

There was a split in people's perceptions of the situation which meant that they were unable to see how it was possible to make up for the effect of the noes. The only hope lay in a shared vision of sufficient richness and depth for

everyone to want to say yes. Civilizations rose on the basis
of such visions, but each in turn flourished and then
declined. Usually they were centred around some concept
similar to the divine right of kings: authority was invested
absolutely in an individual who could do no wrong. Each
time the initial vision and energy came to a peak of
achievement and was unable to sustain that level because of
human divisions.

Gradually there arose groups of people who shared a
vision which was more universal than any authoritarian
vision could ever be. An authoritarian regime denies a
fundamental reality about human nature: that we are
metaphysically one. In absolute terms I am equal with you.
The only way I can get on with you is through a shared
sense of what is required of each of us in the situation we
are in. This involves mutual respect and mutual trust based
on a common spirit which is generous enough to embrace
all surface conflict and differences. The Greeks did this in
developing their acute intellectual and aesthetic sense, and
the Romans in developing justice and order. The Jews went
to the heart of the matter, because they saw that the
fundamental need was for a living integrity in which a
person's circumstances and words and acts were an
indivisible whole. Only this could open the way to
wholeness in the whole human community. There is a
concept in Hebrew of a seamlessness which is experienced as
a unity of action, word and meaning. The prophets
performed seamless acts in which their words were self-
transcendent. This is perhaps the point at which they came
closest to the truth. Yet the Jews still laid the main
emphasis on formal adherence to the law.

The division between inner and outer introduced by the
noes was of a similar nature to the irreconcilability of the
paradoxes which we discussed earlier. We see a similar
pattern today in the apparently irreconcilable attitudes in

the contending factions throughout the world — Ireland and Lebanon for instance. People are locked into history and there is no hope for them within the situation itself. The Greeks could only solve this kind of problem by means of the *Deus ex machina*, a magic wand which sorts everything out. They recognized that there is no way out of such situations via logic.

The impasse could only be broken by an individual who lived out the complete vision to the full: a seamless life in which the current realities of inner and outer were united continuously in someone who was prepared to 'stop the buck' at every level. Mary's life provided an opportunity which was the culmination of centuries of faithful living. She gave birth to a son in whom the sense of the needs of the whole was so complete that his life became a seamless response to his whole experience of it. Christ seized the opportunity, knowing its uniqueness, being aware of the cost and of his own weakness, and holding to his vision of the truth however much appearances seemed to deny it. In doing so he has restored the possibility of wholeness.

# II

---

## FAITHS AND MORALITY

The preceding chapter was concerned with my own sense of the person of Jesus, and to some degree with the Christian religion as a part of the background to my own thinking, as it is now to everyone's to a greater or lesser extent. In the present chapter I would like to move on to a more general discussion of religion and morality. The antagonisms aroused by philosophical debate can be very great, but at least they are generally expressed only at the verbal level: religious antagonisms shed blood. One enters the minefield therefore with great caution.

All religions are concerned with finding the way to wholeness, which is often spoken of as some kind of salvation. Since this is almost by definition the most important aspect of life which one could possibly be concerned with, it is hardly surprising that feeling should run high in this area. Each religion has a different underlying approach to the same goal, and a different history. As a result there are great differences in the formulation of beliefs and in actual practice. The differences can become a matter of life and death, particularly when a religion sees itself as the unique vehicle for the truth.

I would like to set the limits of the word 'religion' as wide as possible. None of the alternatives seems entirely satisfactory. Words such as belief-system or world-view are hardly adequate, because they do not convey the idea of a living body of people and practices. The word church, even with a small c, is too specifically Christian. R.C. Zaehner chose a good phrase in the title of his *Encyclopedia of Living Faiths*, which is a term wide enough to include Dialectical Materialism — though he does not include Science — but 'living faith' is a phrase rather than a word, and 'faith' alone has too many senses.

Science, rationalism, communism, secular humanism and existentialism can all be seen as movements which offer a way of seeing beyond the appearance of the world to its reality, and in that sense they too can properly be called religions. This slightly uncomfortable extension of the meaning of the word is only justified because the proper word does not yet exist. It would be presumptuous to try to invent a word of such wide application, and so all one can do is to take a word which is an example of what one is talking about and use it to stand for the genus to which it belongs. This kind of thing happened, for instance, with the word 'Hoover' (in that case because 'vacuum cleaner' was clumsy), and it is also found in the now embarrassing use of the word 'man' for 'man/woman'. A notorious example is Schopenhauer's use of the word 'will' mentioned in Chapter 9.

The last two examples are, I realize, a warning. The danger is that associations which are normally assumed to apply no longer do so. Normally one links the word 'sacred' with religion, whereas I would like to use the word 'religion' to cover both sacred and secular. This may seem perverse to those who cherish the traditional associations. Its justification is this: it is now vital to recognize that all actual religions in this sense are on the same level. Each is a particular frame of mind writ large, and each has to be treated with equal respect. They are sets of beliefs, attitudes, writings and practices which form the metaphysical source and context of a person's life. What matters is that they are expressions of what individuals care about most deeply in their own particular lives and circumstances: they are the way in which they sense and share the truth of the whole.

The secular/sacred distinction is concerned with outward forms. Jesus drew attention to the balance of secular and sacred when he said, 'Render unto Caesar the things which are Caesar's, and to God the things which are God's.' Since this is an instruction, one is by implication doing right (*ie.* serving God if we wish to put it in those terms) in *both* cases. True religion, whether secular or sacred, is concerned with whether we meet experience in the right spirit whether in the sacred or secular field.

This allows us to see all religions as attempts to express within finite circumstances a truth which potentially embraces them all. In order to illustrate this, I propose to suggest an outline of the development of Christianity which puts it in the context of this wider truth. It is a mistake to think that Jesus came into the world to start another religion. A new religion arose as a result of his coming, but that is quite a different thing. While Christianity contains much that is true we must never identify belief in Jesus with Christendom. What we meet in Jesus and what he said are so revolutionary that it was bound to lead people to preach it and formulate it and teach it. But it is far too universal for any part of society to try to contain it.

If we start with the Early Church, it is quite clear that it began as something of the same nature as the seamless unity mentioned in the previous chapter. From the moment of Pentecost — the third Big Bang — the realization of what the life of Jesus means began to spread into the consciousness of ordinary people. There was initially such an immediate awareness of the truth of the whole situation shared by the disciples that their whole life was a spontaneous activity. We may get a partial insight into this period from some experience of our own where everything seemed to work together of its own accord. When this happens time and space themselves become quite different from our normal experience of them. We become 'absorbed' and 'time flies'; everything is caught up into a wholeness which is intensely present. Temporal and physical proximity to Jesus after the completion of his historical task was clearly accompanied by an astonishing sense of oneness. We can get some idea of this through an imaginative reading of the Acts and Paul's epistles. One senses a quality of combined realism and ecstasy, a complete self-awareness centred on events of the profoundest significance which have actually happened.

There followed a period during which this quality gradually permeated the Ancient World. The Early Fathers established a firm basis for the development of the church's thinking and organization. However the process of diffusion involved the use of other languages than Aramaic. Jesus's words were grounded in the thought-forms of that language and, behind that, of Hebrew. To translate the truth about him and the truth that he taught into Greek and Latin was a task which involved a painful struggle between the very souls of the languages, bound up as each was with a whole way of life and thinking. At the same time there was the associated problem of relating existing patterns of social organization to the new thinking. As a result the first three centuries witnessed a series of sharp conflicts.

When at last Constantine made Christianity the official religion of the Roman Empire there was a strong element of self-contradiction. It became the religion of the majority, and that meant that the Church's role as the vehicle of the gospel was bound to conflict at critical points with its role as one of the powers that be. Augustine's vast theological edifice, nevertheless, was strong enough to survive the violent storms of the Dark Ages.

With the development of Medieval civilization a particular vision of the City of God was brought to fulfilment. The

Christian religion as handed down through the great monastic teachers permeated every aspect of life. Europe to a large extent shared a common culture based on the Church and the Latin language. Thomas Aquinas and others built up the great philosophical system which undergirded the whole medieval culture. The Middle Ages became in turn the foundation for almost everything in the modern world, especially modern languages, science, banking, book-keeping, the modern state. They exhibited many qualities which we need to recover today — especially those that are seen in such vast cooperative activities as the building of the great cathedrals and the creation of their stained glass. There was a common sense of meaningfulness which is still present in the great buildings and institutions which spring from that time.

Nevertheless the Middle Ages were only a staging point. There was still a great deal of pagan influence. Ideas of authority and power were still dominated by ideas prevalent from earliest times. People's thinking was static and literal, in particular their images of the Church, Heaven and Hell, and the City of God. Ideas of right and wrong and the social structure were rigid. The Medieval civilization was far from embodying the fullness of the truth Jesus preached, but it reflected many aspects of that truth, and provided a framework of thought and practice and language which became a womb for the birth of a world civilization.

In England this came to particularly fruitful expression in the trinity of the Book of Common Prayer, the Bible and Shakespeare. The confidence and freshness of the Renaissance often led to great arrogance, but here they were undergirded by the most profound sense of human meaning and love of language. The three books reached deep into people's consciousness. They provided a sound foundation for the development of individual judgment. Ironically this was because the language was so flexible and transparent: it taught people to recognize the taste of the truth, and not to look for the literal truth so mistakenly beloved of fundamentalists. This is what gave these writings their continuing power. They set up a complex web of interrelationships embodying fundamental values which interact at innumerable points with people's lives. They mark the beginning of an age in which Everyman began to think for himself about ultimate issues and make up his own mind instead of accepting what he was told — the age when he became aware of himself as fully responsible.

With the coming of the Reformation and the modern technological and political world we have reached the opposite pole from the time of Jesus. We are at the other end of the spectrum, and can no longer derive literal guidance from what he said. In his time the newness of the message had an impact which is almost impossible for us to imagine now. We have little conception of the general feel of life in those times. Margaret Yourcenar's *Memoirs of Hadrian* gives a glimmering of how it must have felt: it conveys the shut-in feeling experienced even by someone at the top of the tree. Today virtually everybody has come into contact to some extent with people and values directly related to the truth of Jesus, and this makes the situation radically different. The stream of living water has now penetrated physically to almost every corner of the world.

One side of this truth can be found in coming to terms with the world as it is, and not as we would like it to be. This is the great strength of the spirit of reason, as manifested especially in the achievements of science. The personal integrity which underlies all the great discoveries of science is precisely the wholeness which Jesus was talking about when he said 'be perfect'. This kind of honesty and clear-sightedness is the foundation of all the great achievements of civilization, whether in business, science, art, engineering, justice, learning, philosophy or theology.

People talk of the current age as 'Post-Christian', suggesting that we have gone beyond the need for a proper religious understanding of life. That is quite wrong if it is taken to imply that we have gone beyond what Jesus was about. His message has been distorted and smothered all along by the powers that be, and it will continue to be. The story of the Gadarene swine is a clear warning that the cost of healing is immense, and that old ideas exact a terrible toll before they are exorcised. The World Wars, the Stalinist purges, the Holocaust and the Pol Pot massacres are horrifying reminders of the futility of imposing solutions by force. The legacy of each is an appalling psychological trauma which still largely remains to be worked through.

We are under as great a threat as ever. At the same time there are probably more people than ever who are prepared whether they are nominally Christians, Hindus, Muslims, Jews, agnostics or atheists to accept the cost of the integrity which Jesus came to bring. There is a world-wide recognition, particularly among the young, that we need to recover a true human spirituality in our lives. The flower people of the sixties caught this spirit in a touching way, though they were spiritually fragile because largely parasitic. The meditation movement and the interest in Eastern religions, particularly Zen, Buddhism and Hinduism, are another sign of the way people's minds are moving; and so is the growing concern with ecology as a very practical interest in the earth as our common home. All these things are good in their special ways so long as they are a means of relating truly to reality. Each of them also carries a divine health warning: they may be good as means, but there is always the risk that we may be tricked at any moment into treating them as ends in themselves. When that happens we start to worship them as images.

The Old Testament talks of God as jealous. This can upset people, but it is not like human jealousy except that it has to be taken equally seriously. What it means is that the whole structure of reality is highly sensitive to the deeply hidden point at which we turn away from the truth. The betrayal has to be acknowledged and made good as quickly as possible. Each occasion when we let ourselves be tricked into worshipping a cult as an image, regarding it as having absolute authority, is such a point. Both sacred and secular religions lead people to fall into image-worshipping — either physical images such as pictures or objects, or mental images such as dogmas and formulations and theories. This can even apply to the word 'God'. We ignore our sense of the living truth and allow ouselves to be diverted into thinking of objects and ideas as real entities in themselves rather than the outward expression of real relationships.

There is of course a place for distinguishing between sacred and secular. It is a very deep-seated duality, related to the duality between internal and external, possibility and necessity. The outward forms are extremely different, and so for many practical purposes it is right to make the distinction. But 'sacred' must never be automatically identified with 'good'. There must be no easy assumption that the outwardly sacred should always be chosen in preference to the outwardly secular. The sacred certainly points in the direction of unity, because it seeks to arouse a sense of awe, of the need to bring inner and outer into harmony and to cultivate the sensitivity that this requires. The secular is equally necessary because it recognizes that bounds are imposed by the hard facts of the human situation. The struggle between the two at any point should be a struggle to find the way in which the two aspects can be held together without denying the claim of either.

We see something along these lines happening on a global scale between the Superpowers. America seems much more devout and idealistic than Russia, and seems often to believe it has the Divine ear. Russia is cautious about acknowledging religion officially because of the injustices perpetrated in its name and because of its commitment to Communism, but it has a deep seriousness and a concern with things of the spirit which fly in the face of its formal profession. Gorbachov's speeches are often concerned with personal integrity. Both sides have their special contributions to make, and they have to come face to face without fixed ideas about their own rightness.

It is a failure of imagination to look on such a struggle as a zero-sum contest in which if one wins the other must lose. The zero-sum concept is the creation of the imprisoned mind: it is the corollary of conceiving of the situation as finite, with a finite number of options. Situations which are superficially of this kind do exist: we play games which we either win or lose, we set targets which we either achieve or do not achieve, we are involved in litigation and judgment is made either for or against us. But even in these finite situations it is our imaginative attitude and determination that matter. The result matters in that it is a concrete verdict on what happens. But the whole truth includes not only the result but the quality of the efforts on both sides. The greatest games are those in which the result hangs in the balance till the last moment, and in which both sides are raised so far above their expected level that the result becomes secondary.

In an open-ended situation imagination and determination and openness are still more crucial. Ideas happen only when the time and situation and attitudes make it possible for them to happen. We can't force them — as in gardening, the ground has to be prepared and the weather right. The climate is created by a united determination which goes beyond the conscious level. When the time comes ideas spring into being, and it is as if they had been there all the time. The history of ideas is full of examples where different people have had the same ideas at the same time independently. This helps to emphasize that ideas are not the creation of the individual only: they are the product of a great web of acts of faithful attention of which only the last link is forged in the particular person. Ideas for reconciliation especially have to be seen as the product of the whole process, and not of one side or the other.

Morality is an issue almost as fraught as religion. The two are closely connected, more particularly in the great monotheistic religions. Those religions have actually led to a profound misunderstanding of morality, arising from the idea of specific injunctions which must be followed. Jesus corrected this idea but our civilization has barely absorbed what he was saying.

Moral 'laws' are of course far from irrelevant. The Ten Commandments remain as valid as ever as general guides to conduct. There are innumerable cases in which there is no doubt that they indicate the 'right' course. They are based on deep insights and centuries of experience and can never be lightly ignored. But they are not absolute in any simple sense. They are standards which normally apply and which we need good grounds for contravening.

What is in question is where the 'rightness' of an action resides. Is the reason why we should not steal 'because it is a law of God?' If we obey the law simply because we might be caught, is there any merit in that? Nothing significant has been achieved if we do so. If we want to steal and are afraid to, our desire to steal is still there and has not been dealt with. Any choice is 'right' not because the command-ments are intrinsically and automatically right, but because the truth they encapsulate is recognized and accepted to be the truth of the situation. As T.S. Eliot pointed out in *Murder in the Cathedral*,

> The last temptation is the greatest treason:
> To do the right deed for the wrong reason.

The action must be the choice of a free person who recognizes what is required, not the automatic response of a self-satisfied robot.

Blind obedience to rules is a further case of worshipping an image by pre-judging our response. Whenever we do this we cut ourselves off from the truth, replacing responsibility with puppetry. Every proper decision is a free choice in a unique moment in which we trust our own judgment. We have to be ready to follow the truth without any absolute pre-conditions. This does not imply any wilful arbitrariness. Our situation is concrete: we are surrounded by social and intellectual presences which embody centuries of human reflection and experience. These presences help to form our awareness of the true direction of choice.

Simon Gray's acclaimed TV play *After Pilkington* provides a striking case where 'Thou shalt not kill' had to be questioned. He creates a credible situation where an act which the law would describe as murder can not only be defended as morally right in the circumstances, but is actually performed with tenderness and love: death becomes a gift to the 'victim'. Some would argue that even here it was wrong, but that is beside the point: the point is that the person involved was faced with a situation where he could not fall back on an automatic answer — he had to make a courageous decision entirely on his own.

Morality discusses the question of right and wrong largely in terms of our external actions. Jesus went beyond the action to a deeper area, to the choice made internally at the moment of truth. He goes to the heart of the decision, pulling us all up short when he says 'Everyone who looks on a woman lustfully has already committed adultery with her in his heart'. He is not talking about the natural attraction that occurs: there is nothing wrong about that or even about enjoying that. He is talking about the moment in which the soul becomes aware of the idea of making love as a possibility, in complete disregard of all other considerations. At that archetypal point Everyman is aware of a choice. He can either allow the idea to become an obsessively absolute image, or he can accept the idea and bring it into open relationship (within his own mind) to everything and everyone involved. In that timeless moment the critical decision is made: it is the heart of what happens, because it is a yes/no to the full truth of the situation. In that instant it becomes part of the structure of things.

Some people would see this as a difficult and perhaps even foolish attempt at self-control, but I have not said anything about whether the desire for the person should be pursued. Natural desire forms a starting point for relationships. The question is whether the desire, the moment it is experienced, becomes an image which for that very reason separates us from the reality of the other person, or whether it is brought into relationship with the other person as a person. This is not psychologically damaging or impossible. One way in which a man can do this — as was suggested once to me by someone of profound human understanding — is to use his imagination to visualize his sexual power spreading through the body to the extremities to link to the whole world. Instead of being hypnotically concentrated in one focal point it then lifts the whole body into an open and sensitive relationship to everything. For a woman the idea of power might be replaced by the dual idea of longing, but the same idea would apply: the longing to embrace reality would extend and be felt throughout the body. For both sexes wide openness and sensitivity are central.

The really testing case comes when it is a matter not of simple lust but of true love in conflict with convention. True love is essentially holistic and so is intimately bound up with the body. This is the kind of experience out of which great literature and drama are made. They involve us in turning points on a cosmic stage where the individual has to wrestle with her own truth, make her own choice, and live or die with the decision. Drama helps us to use imaginative insight to get to the heart of the action, and so brings home to us the need for each of us to face the truth. The scale may seem much smaller, but our decisions are of the same kind and are equally of eternal significance. There is another parallel with the world of drama: moments are like theatre seats — if they are not filled at the time they are lost for ever.

At the beginning of this chapter we found a gap in our language: there was no single word which would cover everything we wanted to, combining the idea of vision, community, creed and practice. This suggests that people are not yet able to see them as a single category comprising a whole spectrum of members. The unitary word does not exist, and so any word used tends to split people into mutually exclusive camps.

I have suggested that Jesus did not primarily come to found a religion, or for that matter to preach a morality in the sense of laying down universal commandments. The two great commandments are concerned not with what we do but with the spirit in which we live. We are indoctrinated with the idea that Jesus has to be identified with Christianity. This leads us to take it for granted that a response to him automatically requires allegiance to the Church in some form and adherence to so-called Christian principles. The true Christly tradition (*ie.* that which is concerned not primarily with the historic link to Jesus but with his reality) respects the vehicles which are the means by which many aspects of the truth reach us, but it always asks in each situation 'Where is Jesus in this?' without making any automatic assumptions. One of my goddaughters visiting the Rock in Jerusalem was struck by the fact that the church was dark, elaborate and gloomy, while the mosque was spacious, simple and full of light. Which is nearer to Jesus?

It is ironic that an organization has grown up described as Jesus's Body which says that it can offer salvation if we conform to its teaching and practices. This is the same kind of offer as was made by the Pharisees. They offered the reward of being seen to be righteous and the prosperity that could be expected to go with it. The Church offers the image of eternal bliss. The High Churchman says, 'Perform this practice and be saved', the Low Churchman or the evangelist says, 'believe (according to some formula) and be saved'. Both risk diverting attention from real salvation to the idea of something guaranteed. The message of Jesus was surely, 'There is no guarantee except choosing to be with me in the present, sharing it fully with everyone.' There is nothing here we can claim as our own. We simply open ourselves to his truth, the truth of the whole within us, allowing it to work freely in us so that we are the truth where we are. What we find in ourselves may be ridiculous or comic or terrifying: it is all a reflection of the whole. We have to meet it in trust at the point where we know that the questioning, for the moment, has to stop.

This helps us to get the question of other religions into perspective. Christianity has always tended to claim that it is the unique truth, because of the uniqueness of Jesus. When it was first proclaimed it was quite clear that the self-awareness of Christians was far beyond the limited vision of the people who were converted: it came as a revelation whose impact now is difficult to conceive. The truth of the gospel was self-authenticating and its impact for many pagans was overwhelming. The famous story that Bede tells about the missionary Paulinus preaching to King Edwin of Northumbria is worth repeating as a reminder of this. After Paulinus had spoken, one of the king's chief men (unnamed) said:

> 'Your majesty, when we compare the present life of man with that time of which we have no knowledge, it seems to me like the swift flight of a lone sparrow through the banqueting hall where you sit in the winter months to dine with your thanes and counsellors. Inside there is a comforting fire to warm the room; outside, the wintry storms of snow and rain are raging. This sparrow flies swiftly in through one door of the hall, and out through another. While he is inside, he is safe from the winter storms; but after a few moments of comfort, he vanishes from sight into the darkness whence he came. Similarly, man appears on earth for a little while, but we know nothing of what went before this life, and what follows. Therefore if this new teaching can reveal any more certain knowledge, it seems only right that we should follow it.'

Today Christianity is only one of several major religions in a world whose self-awareness has been awoken. There are still many needs which it is uniquely able to provide, and it alone provides the unbroken personal link with Jesus himself through history. It continues to wrestle with the theological and practical problems of faith. It maintains an environment of worship and devotion in which the kernel of truth can be passed from one generation to the next. As much as any religion it has a particular compassion for the poor, sick and underprivileged, and it proclaims the truth that every person is of equal absolute worth. This vision is the root of the care and concern shown in our society.

But the kernel is Jesus, and his presence in the world is more like the great tree that he spoke of in which all those who love the truth can have their nest. The knowledge of Jesus has spread throughout the world both consciously and unconsciously, and goes far beyond any attempt to confine it. Each person and each religion has had to absorb and relate to his truth in its own way. The gospel includes the message that the preachers need the listeners as much as *vice versa*. Each religion, including the secular ones, has its own special light to bring.

One 'sacred' religion has grown up since Christianity which incorporates some key elements of Jesus's message and in many ways comes very close to his spirit. Islam teaches the unity of all things under Allah and thus preaches a profound egalitarianism: even though it allows polygamy, for instance, it insists that all the children are to be treated equally. Like the monasteries it makes practical provision for a rhythmic alternation between inner and outer, worship and action, which reconciles those basic dualities. Its message that every detail matters is very close to that of Jesus.

It is obvious that people of other religions exhibit deep awareness of the truth. Any attempt by Christians to claim that they are the sole possesors of 'The Truth' is in itself self-defeating: it derives from ideas of authority which Jesus himself sought to overturn. Christians are particular people with a particular background and a particular history. The same is true of those of other religions. These are facts which are themselves part of the situation in which we meet: they are differences which have to be lived through, but the starting-point is the recognition that each of us is equally a centre of self-awareness, and that everything of worth springs from our faithfulness to that. Where there are disagreements they are evidence that the truth has not yet been reached, and it has to be sought in a spirit of equality and generosity and acceptance of pain.

Once the nature of self-awareness has been recognized — that it seeks to reconcile itself to itself through free choice of the truth — the question of religious practice and loyalty falls into place. There is no objection to preaching in order to give the good news to those who have not heard it, but

the idea of notching up converts is anathema to the spirit of
Jesus. It is right to seek to safeguard the truth, but it has
grown to maturity now and is strong enough to transcend
disagreements. One can no longer identify those who are 'on
the right side' by their declared loyalty. Each of us moves
from the right side to the wrong side from moment to
moment according to the way we face the immediate truth.
In this situation it is no longer a matter of gathering the
saved into the ark. We need to strengthen each other so
that our linked awareness becomes a transforming and
enlivening power which catches everyone and everything up
into a minutely differentiated whole to which all contribute
their share.

The idea of a heaven and hell *after* death is misconceived.
It arises out of medieval ideas of time and space involving a
temporal concept of the soul. These lead us to think in
terms of individual damnation in crude physical terms.
Salvation or damnation is always in the present: the proper
basic unit is not the person but the person-moment. At
every moment we are eternally damned or saved according
as we respond yes or no to what the moment offers. Each of
us is judged in each moment: each — even the 'hard of
heart' — moves from heaven to hell and back, and has no
guarantee beyond trusting. To recognize that is to recognize
our common plight.

The Christian tradition is not to be dismissed, but rather
broadened. Jesus did not brush aside his own tradition. He
loved it and cherished it, and welcomed it as a basis on
which to build. He used it to get across the truth about
people — not about the Jews only, but about the whole
world and its relation to its own truth. For the most part
there was no reason why he should separate himself from
the synagogue: it was tending in the same direction and
carried on the teaching of Moses and the spirit of the
prophets. The division only came when the Jews realized

that he was going too far for comfort below the surface of established orthodoxy to the reality on which it was founded. They were dismayed when he faced them with that truth, showing them that the very nature of truth is that it must be freely chosen at each point, and that he was prepared to live out the implications of this to their ultimate conclusion.

# 12

## FULFILMENT

This book is a search for a basis for understanding. One could write endlessly about the topics raised, but at this stage there is nothing to be gained by going into too much detail. Enough has been said to provide an outline, and it is time to sum up and to set out the implications.

The book by J.B. Phillips entitled *Your God is too small* seized on a cardinal point. Our conception of God, or reality, or whatever we wish to call the whole, is often pitifully cramped and weak. We imagine that if we have discovered and confirmed the relatively simple patterns discernible in the physical world, or gained insight into the workings of the human mind, we have mastered the mystery. We imagine that knowledge is power, and that we can use it to manipulate people or things or events. We have little sense of the unfathomable truth that everything is a perfectly integrated expression of all that we are.

There is the dual truth that we are all that reality can be at the point where we are. We cannot be forced to acknowledge reality, and often it seems that we lack the strength or ability or will to do so. We can only seek to sense the longing which was made most fully manifest in the life of Jesus, and to develop the feeling that the truth is waiting for us to become aware of it and embrace it. There can be no certainty: the only guarantee is trust on every side, and this includes trust that reality will keep its side of the bargain. It seems an impossible dream, and yet many who have most reason to doubt it know that it is not. It is the only position which is intellectually tenable, whatever the surface appearances to the contrary, and it is vital that we should recognize this. It is becoming more and more obvious how threadbare the old ideas of power and military might and ruthless competition have become. All the old idealisms and realisms have been tried and have eventually been found wanting. Yet we still hanker after these solutions, as if they could ever provide a guarantee of Utopia.

After two thousand years of thought and study about the words and life of Jesus we still for the most part have a badly distorted conception of their meaning and significance. He is still far more revolutionary than any of us can really imagine. We try to explain to ourselves what he said and did, using comforting and familiar categories like love, goodness, justice and mercy, and we easily forget that though these terms may sometimes convey a sense of the inner reality that Jesus was talking about, they can never *be* that reality. We talk about Jesus's ethical teaching, of his demand for the renunciation of the world, of his emphasis on the inner motive, and we still do not get to the real point. He was going far beyond saying 'if you do this you will be all right, you will have your reward in heaven', or 'you will build a healthy society'. Every word that he uttered was simply the expression of his awareness of what was needed at that moment, and it was all one with his ultimate message 'The Kingdom of God is upon you' and its dual 'The Kingdom of God is within you'.

Because of its authoritarian and theistic associations the phrase 'Kingdom of God' is archaic now. Jesus was speaking universally, in a climate where it was more difficult for people to think universally than it is now: that is part of the reason why he was not properly understood. We live in a world which is physically one in a way which goes far beyond even what I knew as a child: people on opposite sides of the world can interact directly with ease. There is indeed the conceivable possibility that we might be able to interact with beings in space, but to look seriously to that for salvation is escapism. For all practical purposes we are on our own, and that is the reality we have to live with: a single world which presents what we are to ourselves.

The major difference between the Kingdom of God and many religious programmes is that it is based on a living awareness of the whole of reality centred around the present moment. Jesus does not lay upon us impossible pre-defined requirements. He does not expect that we shall reach perfection by observing a single lofty code. Codes of behaviour are part of our knowledge, and they must be taken into account, but they do not touch the essence of what Jesus was and is saying. He addresses each of us simultaneously and says, 'Here you are, at this particular place, at this particular time, in this particular situation. What is happening to you, what you enjoy or suffer, what thoughts or ideas occur, who you are with, what you see and hear and smell and taste and feel, what you have experienced and know, are all a presentation to you of the human state as it relates to you now. You know that each of your fellows is experiencing his own situation in his own way: you know about some directly, you know by hearsay of others, you know there is a great multitude who are there but beyond any possibility of direct knowledge. Each of you is a gateway for awareness of the truth to enter the world. All that you are asked to do is to seek that awareness openly and to say yes to what you recognize needs to be done.'

This is a translation of 'Love the Lord your God with all your heart, with all your soul, with all your mind', the universal commandment which applies everywhere and always. Since it is universal it cannot be specific in any material sense: it is specific only in saying that you are asked to face the truth of your specific circumstances.

Our seeking has to be deliberate, critical and open. If it is genuine there can be a deeply hidden rightness which can be sensed inwardly but need rarely be expressed. Nor need the doing be an external act: it may simply mean turning inwardly to grapple with and embrace the reality we are faced with. The purest form in which this happens is in prayer or meditation. Prayer is not asking directly for specific things, apart from articulating the fact that we have a natural human desire for them. It is the inner self opening up to reality, and being prepared to embrace the cost of that whatever it is. Since this is such a pure exercise of choice the way in which it is reflected in what happens will go far beyond what we expect.

This can all sound like one more impossible ideal unless we recognize that in practice there is a continual movement between the most humdrum state and the most extreme crisis points, and between the deepest depression and the greatest elation. What we are asked to do is not to pretend that these are not there, not to imagine that they are justly deserved punishments or rewards, but to recognize that each state presents us with the work that is needed now. When we are hemmed in, the work is to wait and watch; when the way ahead presents itself, we take it. The readiness and openness are everything.

The ancient and medieval civilizations took a human-centred view of the universe. They found the source of meaning in the king, the emperor, the god, the Father-figure God 'out there'. This view was rudely shaken by Copernicus, and still further undermined by Darwin and Freud. Copernicus showed that the physical centre of our system was the sun, and the earth a mere satellite; Darwin portrayed us as part of the evolutionary process with adaptation and survival as our goal; Freud showed that we had much less control over ourselves than we had thought. These ideas forced us to abandon our view of ourselves as lords of creation, as well as any anthropomorphic view of God. They were a great psychological shock which a lot of people have still not got over. They performed a service in stripping away our illusions, but also carried away much that was of great value. They are very partial views of our true position.

It is time for a fresh view of things, and a new reformation. We are neither the masters nor the puppets of creation: the Bible rightly calls us stewards. At the moment most of us are confused stewards: so much seems to have gone wrong, there are so many villains roaming free, the United Nations has its hands tied, the mature nations are still preoccupied with gaining an ever higher standard of living and an ever larger share of the world's wealth. We are surrounded on all sides by the clamour of the media and the cheerful shouts of the barrow boys of commerce and the conflicting pronouncements of experts. We can no longer believe in making any real headway by conscious indoctrination and manipulation.

Proper education and thought and political activity are necessary, but they derive their strength entirely from the real source of all worth — free choice. This is far deeper than any superficial political concept, which too easily becomes a matter of having the money to spend as you like, and too easily ignores the fact that the plight of others is part of the subject matter of choice. Renewal comes about when each individual seeks the truth and chooses it at the intersection of conscious and unconscious at which he recognizes it. That is the sole point at which wholeness can enter.

Holography is a scientific technique which allows us to create a three-dimensional representation of an object through the interference patterns from two sources of light which are stored on film. A remarkable property of the hologram is that if we split the film into pieces, each piece contains enough information to reconstitute the object. This provides an illustration of the nature of our experience. Each of us stands at the meeting point of outer and inner worlds, and each of us is like a fragment of a hologram: the whole picture is present in each of us. This analogy treats the hologram as a metaphor for the unity of the individual and the whole.

There is a dual interpretation of this analogy, as a metaphor for our experiences as they are presented to us. A hologram creates the appearance of a solid object through interference patterns so that the observer 'sees' a three-dimensional body. Without the aid of other senses (assuming there are no detectable blemishes) he would not be able to distinguish it from the actual solid body. The idea of the hologram brings us closer to the way things actually work than the idea of objects which are in some mysterious way 'out there'. The hologram of real life creates an appearance which is realistic to all the senses. It can be understood as a precise representation in the present moment of the interference patterns generated by our individual relationships with each other and with the whole structure. It is not something which is 'real' in an absolute sense: it is the *product* of reality.

We are aware of being aware, of being each a centre of presence which is related to every other such centre. It is this self-awareness which is the ground of everything. Its nature requires a complete self-consistency so that every facet of our internal experience is precisely related to every facet of our external experience. The only dimension in which anything real can happen is the dimension of choice. Each act of choice is then reflected back to us in the relationship between our feelings, our concepts and our external experience.

At each instant each of us is free to be or not to be the truth. This sounds extremely simple. The simplicity was underlined by Jesus when he said:

My yoke is good to bear, my load is light,

and by T.S. Eliot in *Four Quartets*:

Quick now, here, now, always —
A condition of complete simplicity
(Costing not less than everything).

But the 'everything' that is required can take every conceivable form, and the illusion of fragmentation can sometimes be so powerful that it seems impossible to avoid its hypnotic effect. Every moment presents a new pattern, and we may allow ourselves to be deceived into thinking that we are powerless to deal with the endless proliferation. Ironically we are powerless as long as we imagine that we have to exercise control in some manipulative way based on our past knowledge. The way to freedom is to recognize that we are presented not only with the situation but with the means of transfiguring the situation by allowing reality to enter it completely. It always seems impossible till we do it, and then it is simple. The key — and the cost — lies in the determination to look beyond the seeming.

This may sound individualistic. Western thought is dominated by the idea of the individual, and the concept of the primacy of the individual conscience is one of its cornerstones. There are occasions when everyone else refuses to acknowledge the truth of the situation and only one person is willing or able to do so. Our high valuation of the individual is based on our recognition that on such occasions it is essential that he should hold on, because the well-being of the whole depends on it.

At the same time the truth of the situation is the truth for everyone involved, and unless the individual is holding onto *this* truth, his firmness becomes obstinacy. There is often a common wisdom which reflects the truth more faithfully than any individual does. Napoleon may have been the only person who could see his star, but he knew he had to get his people to share the sense that the star was there and was real. It is from this shared awareness that any achievements come. Jesus saw further than any star and reached to the reality of the whole. When this vision is linked to our common awareness all things are possible.

It is the fashion today to pay lip service to wholeness. But much of our talk is still in the language of historical and social processes, in terms of laws and forces and power. Science is spoken of as if it is wresting secrets from nature; politically minded people seek to reach positions of power and influence; the earth is still largely regarded as something to be exploited. These attitudes continue to be infected with old ways of thinking and talking and writing, and they distort our perception. Our goal must be a true understanding of the cosmos, a true root sense. There is one reality in which everything is related. This is the plain truth of the matter: what each of us chooses to call this reality matters in particular contexts but is essentially secondary. Each of us need be neither an automatic programmed creature nor a soul longing to escape from the flesh, but can seek to be reality fully present in the unique context, linking the inner and outer worlds.

We can see the world we experience as the presentation of our total state. Its characteristic forms are twofoldness in relation to finite entities such as objects and classes, and threefoldness in relation to infinities such as persons. Space and time themselves are not absolutes, but are categories which are appropriate for relating experiences to each other. The absolute categories are the infinite unity of self-awareness and the null multiplicity of the forms of our relationships. The true centre of everything is the eternal now, around which our finite experience dances in a flux without beginning and without end but with intent, meaning and worth. It is what Eliot in *Four Quartets* called

> . . . the still point of the turning world.

There is a natural web linking each individual situation to the heart of reality, from the particular to the universal. There is no visible centre of authority from which true judgment emanates hierarchically and is implemented through simple acts of obedience. The true view is that each individual is linked into the whole on the basis of equal worth, and authority arises at the point which is appropriate for the situation.

As we move from particular to universal we do not move 'higher' in any real sense. Civilization tends to encourage this idea because the people at the top easily convince themselves that they are more important. Certainly their decisions have a more wide-ranging effect, certainly they are better educated, probably they have a wider and deeper insight into the processes within society. But their worth has nothing to do with these factors. It has everything to do with the spirit which informs their decisions, and this lies deep in the way in which they meet each choice. If they take the true view, they will recognize that the critical link with reality can appear at any level, and will be prepared to welcome any contribution if it connects with the truth.

It is this inner spirit, this attitude to the whole, which is the crucial element of each human situation. We detect it in each other in innumerable subtle ways. A simplified idea of it appears in the idea of motive, but that can put too much emphasis on the particular conscious aim. Ideas of incorruptibility and personal integrity come much nearer. It is a question of whether we hold on like grim death to part of ourselves or the world, or are willing to be critically open to the eternal newness with which we are surrounded, and to face it fully.

To view things in this way reverses our normal perception of everything. It provides a global context in which we can see that meaning is possible at the deepest level, even though there are times when we dare not utter the thought. The meaning itself is self-transcendent, not dependent on any external proof or certainty: it is real because the belief in the meaning is grounded in reality. It is the heart of what we perceive as true worth.

There is still confusion in people's minds about the nature of belief. It is frequently contrasted with the idea of scientifically established fact. Scientists sometimes speak as if people's beliefs are illusions even though they work — for instance in healing. This kind of talk turns language on its head: the scientists themselves are under the illusion that facts have a reality which the beliefs do not. The plain truth is that every scientific fact derives its standing from belief, and it is the belief itself which is the reality on which science is built. Objectivity lies in open, honest and questioning belief. It cannot be finally expressed but only sensed and known directly.

The idea of explanation also needs widening. We tend to think in terms of cause and effect, and to base our explanations on past experience, and on analogies with other situations. This eventually results in either circularity or infinite regress, like dictionary definitions, unless it ends in the judgment 'Yes, I'm prepared to accept that is true' by a human being. The real explanation can only be in terms of the whole, and so may seem unattainable. We can however have a conception of it: the universal explanation is that what happens is a continuous and precise interaction between all that is, all that has been and all that can be — both internal and external — taking all the implications into account. All scientific laws and all moral laws are abstractions from the experience of this.

Though this is no detailed explanation, it clears the ground so that we can begin to understand things in principle. It recognizes that we are continuously presented with experiences which are the precise response of reality — love — to the whole human state, past, present and future. It is impossible for us to imagine how this comes about, but it is possible to conceive of it and to have a sense of its intellectual coherence. We can even conceive that the response itself is a kind of act of faith along the lines of an artist's trust in the potential integrity of the whole work while it is as yet incomplete. We can sense and trust that this is so.

Belief is central; not an expressed belief in a formulation, but pure belief in the worth and reality of believing. It is love in each individual reaching out to love as it sustains the whole fabric of creation. But it is no easy belief that all our wishes will come true: the belief is always subject to the conditions inherent in the particular situation. These present us with the reality of all that has happened, and we must pay detailed attention if our belief is to be focused.

The word 'holiness' has become devalued: such phrases as 'holier-than-thou' associate it with a kind of piety which is ultimately arrogant and proud. The idea behind the word is perhaps too potent for modern people to be comfortable with: it suggests an intensity and seriousness which are hard for people to take. But it still carries a sense of the general attitude we need to cultivate. As far as external behaviour is concerned it can go with both seriousness and light-heartedness. It means a deep reverence for the reality of every aspect of our life, and a determination to embrace even the darkest and most sordid and most tedious sides so that wholeness may fill them.

We live in the context of a fulfilment which is both unguaranteed and possible. The nature of the fulfilment is quite different from the sort of progress (not to be spurned, but kept in proportion) which nineteenth century idealists sought. It lies not in winning knowledge and manipulating our environment, but in opening the way for true worth to fill the fabric of the world. There are two metaphors which are particularly appropriate here: the metaphor of filling out to completeness, and the metaphor of matching so that inner and outer complement each other in a perfect harmony — like the stability achieved by perfect balance. We can relate these to the pattern of the cross. The filling is in the vertical dimension, where nothingness is completely filled with spirit, and the matching or balance is in the horizontal dimension where Yin and Yang embrace in perfect union.

Our traditional modes of thought hanker after absolutes which we can hang onto physically and which provide a guarantee of correctness. These modes lie at the root of dogmatism, fundamentalism and superstition. They are always, however disguised, an attempt to escape from facing the immediate concreteness of the present situation, and from allowing the fullness of love to enter it and transform it. There are many who imagine that their interest lies in maintaining and fostering such absolutism. They build images for people to worship — not only obviously false images such as the Third Reich or Bible-belt fundamentalism, but the most august creations of our civilization (the law, science, church and state) and the highest ideals (freedom, equality, even the sanctity of life). These are worthy of the greatest respect, but at the same time must be viewed continually in the light of the truth. Wherever they are used to manipulate people's minds and to deceive people into treating them as absolute, worth is undone and the fabric of the universe is torn. Love is the only absolute, the only guarantee of freedom and worth.

The practical requirements of love can fluctuate from moment to moment, because they depend on the choices that are made as they are made. A choice is made in a realm beyond everything we observe and feel, and it cannot be pre-determined. Many today lament the loss of

absolute standards of right and wrong. This is a false
nostalgia. There always has been and always is an absolute
right and wrong: it consists in accepting or denying love as
it seeks to fill the moment. The outward form of what we
'should' do is inherently ambiguous right up to the point
where we actually choose. The choice alone can incarnate
the truth. Before the decision we consider arguments on one
side and on the other. Both will generally have force, and
we may feel ourselves caught in a dilemma which presents
itself as the choice between evils. The whole worth of the
decision consists in bringing all our imagination to bear to
avoid the evils, and in recognizing when the choice has to
be made. We have to watch for the feeling within the bones
that it is time to choose, and then base our choice on our
inner knowledge of the right course.

It may then appear to have been a terrible mistake, so
that the worth of the decision appears to be nullified. We
have trusted and apparently been let down. Here is one of
the hardest of all situations to face: it can destroy confidence
and lead to disillusion. It has to be tackled at the roots by
recognizing it as a deception. We are being tempted to
judge the worth of the decision by its results. If we do this
we judge the infinite by the finite, and so deny the very
heart of the fundamental truth.

Of course if things go wrong it is a message to us that we
need to find out why: the experience and the knowledge
gained from it becomes part of the background to future
choices. But the lie we are tempted to succumb to is that
the yes which we said to our deepest sense of what was right
was of no worth. On the contrary it is a seed of eternal
worth implanted in that moment, and the fact that things
'went wrong' is a sign of the deep disharmony which still
remains to be resolved. The experience of failure when we
know we chose rightly is a great personal price to pay. To
accept its cost with neither bitterness nor hopeless acquies-

cence throws the door wide open for reality to enter.

That is what the Bible describes in the Book of Job. Job's only comfort lay in his positive acceptance that his apparently undeserved suffering was God's will. There can be no direct link between an individual's goodness and his success: this would be trivial and pointless, and would in the end separate one person from the other. The link is the other way round: the deeper the person's faith, the greater the burden of disharmony he can be entrusted with. But only real life can do the entrusting, because it must take into account everything that is involved. The link has to extend all the way from the individual's choice to the integrity of the whole.

There is no room for making comparisons in this respect. Judgments of the depth of a person's faith are to be avoided above all. In human terms it is possible to talk of a person's faith growing, and we can look upon that as a kind of spiritual potential embodied in the whole physical make-up of the person, both mental and bodily. But the parable of the labourers in the vineyard is a reminder that there is always the same reward to be earned, and the only condition for earning it is to do what is necessary when we are faced with it. The only 'reward' we can expect is the awareness that we are saying yes when it is needed. This is the same for everyone, and it is simply a delight in being one with truth and with those who are facing the truth. This may not always be an unalloyed pleasure, but there are deeper springs of fulfilment than that.

All things are possible, but only when everyone says yes. Human logic says that there is no possibility whatsoever of this happening: life simply goes on and on in time, with people living and suffering and dying, with the world getting fuller and fuller and the earth being exploited more and more, until either we destroy ourselves or run out of resources. The logic of reality presents a quite different picture. It says that the things we experience are the direct and exact expression of the state we are in, which is determined by the real pattern of our yeses and noes and our present knowledge of them and relationship to them.

The sense that the response is precise, that reality continually presents events and ideas and feelings which are perfectly matched to each particular moment, assures us of the intellectual coherence of our attitude. It is of the very nature of love that it has to do justice to nothingness, and incorporate the 'evil' and the missed opportunities of the noes into the fabric of the universe without waving a magic wand. All the constraints of continuity and formal integrity have to be observed. The only consistent way in which inner and outer can be truly matched is through individuals recognizing the necessary cost and having the courage to embrace it. Each time this happens the meaning of the whole is created afresh.

The response of reality is incredibly delicate and subtle, far beyond the sensitivity of our very greatest artists and composers and poets and thinkers. It respects each of our noes, and will only act within the bounds that they impose, and will only move 'forward' as it is given the opportunity of our yeses. The yeses, the faith, of the people of Israel provided the opportunity for love to enter fully into the heart of things in Jesus. The logic of a true belief in him, not to be confused with a belief in formal Christianity, though certainly consistent with true Christianity and true Judaism and true Islam and true Hinduism and true Buddhism as well as true reason and true communism and true humanism, is to trust that his continuous yes embodied in a single whole life is a seed which can fill the whole of our life. Just as his continuous yes was an impossibility which we can nevertheless sense as real, so the filling of the universe with a joint simultaneous yes *seems* an impossibility which we can nevertheless *choose to believe* to be within the real bounds of what is possible.

The physical notion of reality is simply a special aspect of reality on which we have concentrated disproportionately over the last few centuries. The meaning of 'real' goes far beyond that. It points to a relationship between inner and outer which is completely whole, which respects the facts, which catches up every smallest detail into a living unity. Lovers who experience the heights of human love have a foretaste of such fullness: the whole space in which they dwell is transformed, and time is suspended. Saints and mystics have a similar foretaste in their communion with God. Leaders and athletes and artists at the height of their powers know something of what it is like. The glimpse of the formal and real perfection of everything which I experienced was of the same kind. Simple joy and laughter spring from the same root. Everyone has some experience, however apparently minor, of the unutterably true. For all of us the glimpses such as they are are partial: they come unbidden, and leave us with the sense of possibility. They are signs of wholeness, but are not to be consciously sought as a guarantee of our own delight. Ecstasy can be catastrophically divisive unless it is shared.

Such experiences can seem divorced from reality because of the current state of things, and once they have passed, the contrast of ordinary life can seem to deny their worth and validity. Within them our only wish is that they should go on for ever, and when they have passed we long to recover the state. But what we experience in them is reality in its fullness, we experience our true self which is love, and love requires us to venture out and join with everyone else in finding reality together. The choice between appearance and what we know to be reality confronts us all continuously, taking ever-changing forms but constant in its challenge. While time itself is the condition of our lives we can have no certainty: everything hangs in the balance in each moment, and everything depends on the faith of each one of us. We are asked to make each choice in deliberate, passionate, imaginative sanity, in awareness of what love is saying to us in each now, in hope of the impossible miracle of transformation. You ask, 'Can this really happen?' Yes — the moment we each choose freely to say yes.

# PART TWO

# FOURFOLD FORM

# CONTENTS

## 1. INTRODUCTION

This paper can be seen as a dual of Part I. It offers a different perspective, summarizing the main philosophical ideas and developing them into a more formal model. For some this is not needed: they see through intuitively to the truth that I am trying to express. The paper is for those who like myself seek intellectual coherence and feel the need for ideas to be set out in philosophical form.

For convenience I shall refer to the model by the acronym ASIF. This relates to the title for Part I, and it also stands for 'Alternative Shared Intellectual Framework'.

## 2. THE EINSTEINIAN SHIFT

We grow up with the idea of absolute laws, expressed in forms of words such as the Ten Commandments, or in ideas of absolute love and truthfulness. From these we derive prescriptions for the way in which we should behave. We conceive that for each defined situation there is some predetermined ideal which all right-thinking people would expect us to seek to acheve.

For some purposes this suffices, but it is only a crude guide, and it leads to destructive fundamentalism if taken as the universally right approach to the human situation. It leads to wrong decisions in critical cases. The difference between this traditional view and the ASIF resembles the difference between the Newtonian view of the physical universe and the Einsteinian view. In Newton's scheme the laws are absolute, but apply for no reason other than that they apply. For Einstein the laws arise out of the geometry of space-time: they express the implications of self-consistency. It is harder for us to understand them in detail, but the quality of explanation is correspondingly deeper. It gets closer to what is really going on, and transforms our attitude to it.

The practical difference between the two views may seem

small, only revealed by critical experiments. The metaphysical difference is total, because it is the difference between an absolute Cartesian view of the universe as something 'out there' and a view which recognizes that the observer is an integral part of our conception. The Newtonian system, beautiful as it is, is ultimately closed, once-for-all, take-it-or-leave it, and places the observer in a position of aloof detachment. The Einsteinian view is open, and acknowledges that even deeper insights may be reached through human exchange and involvement.

Einstein shows that our description of the physical world depends on our position and speed. Quantum Mechanics shows that it depends on our choice of relative precision for velocity and position. The observer is inextricably involved in the facts. That does not mean that the facts are any less real, but it puts everything onto a completely different metaphysical basis. This pioneering imaginative achievement of science has been repeated in many other fields. It is a recognition that nothing is real in the sense of being 'out there' absolutely independently of everything else.

The Newtonian view is brilliantly simple but leads to great intellectual and metaphysical distortions and problems. Similarly metaphysics based purely on logical argument and on absolute forms is relatively clearcut but leads to profound difficulties in our thinking. There is no way in which we can pre-define what is 'right' for a situation in terms of some pre-existent form on the basis of a carefully structured logical argument. That would be like Nanny telling us to obey 'because I say so'. A choice is right not because it expresses obedience to some prescription but because it is right in the light of the whole situation at the very moment in which it is made. The absoluteness of what is right is real enough, but it is inextricably bound up with the uniqueness of the situation.

## 3. KINDS OF FACT

While Wittgenstein said that we must be silent about those things whereof we cannot speak, he also suggested that those things are more important than the things we can speak of. The Logical Positivists and their successors, however, have done their best to see that they are relegated to the status of nonsense and so by implication worthless. We are therefore taught to split facts into only two basic categories: verifiable physical facts such as 'there is a squirrel in the garden', and formal facts such as '$2 + 2 = 4$'. This is standard philosophic practice, and it is reinforced by the dominance of the scientific approach which is concerned only with observable facts.

The result is that facts about the inner world are not normally accorded their proper status: they are relegated to the secondary status of 'subjective'. Yet to have an idea or to have toothache or to like Mozart are undeniable facts which have just as much influence on our relationship to life as facts of the first two kinds. They are an integral part of the structure of reality.

Each of us is largely on her own in relation to inner facts. They are not accessible to the public realm. This and other factors contribute to the root imbalance in our conception of life which arises from our down-grading of inner facts. In practice we believe that they are of great importance, but if our expressed ideas do not tie in with our practice and with reality, disaster lies in wait.

We need a proper conception of the way in which facts of our individual inner worlds relate to facts in our common outer world. Attempts to cope with this problem in simple mechanistic ways have failed. The whole idea of simple causality which is so effective in the physical sciences is useless when trying to link mental and physical experiences, because it is not appropriate for the realm of subjectivity. A causality operates, but not in this simple form.

## 4. BASIC CATEGORIES

The pattern of the cross described in Chapter 3 of Part I provides a more appropriate way of thinking of the different kinds of fact. It displays the four fundamental categories: infinite, outer, inner, zero. The last three correspond to physical facts, personal facts and formal facts. The first (infinite) corresponds to the single fact of the reality of the whole.

This pattern provides a basic set of dimensions — *ie.* modes in which we can interpret and share our experience. We can think of the body of facts in each dimension as constituting its own apparently independent world. So we can begin with the following basic picture:

World 1  Physical (outer) facts      (in Dimension 1)
World 2  Personal (inner) facts      (in Dimension 2)
World 3  Formal (conceptual) facts (in Dimension 3)

To these we need to add an ultimate dimension, which represents the reality in which the three dimensions are finally related. It is like the origin in a set of geometric axes and like zero in the set of integers: we accept that it is meaningful even though we cannot say exactly what it is. So there is a fourth dimension:

World 0  Reality as a whole      (in Dimension 0)

The most useful dimensions are those which ensure that facts in one dimension are as far as possible independent of facts in the others. The set described above goes a long way towards satisfying that criterion, but there is nothing absolute about it. It is simply a useful way of organizing our thinking and examining our use of language. It embodies a pattern which recurs in experience again and again. We can think of all our experiences as presentations of reality (World 0) via Worlds 1, 2 and 3. Rearranging the pattern, we can see ourselves each as a node (*) standing at the meeting point of the four worlds:

```
    0                    Reality
  2 * 1          Inner    *    Outer
    3                     Form
```

This is a kind of metaphysical atom, a fourfold pattern at the heart of our experience. Like a physical atom it is a form we can detect in what is going on: it has no absolute reality in itself. We can recognize it at every level. Here are four examples:

| Living | Sexual | Mathematical | Logical |
|---|---|---|---|
| Presence | Love | Infinity | All |
| Personal * Physical | Female * Male | $-1$ * $+1$ | Or * And |
| Necessity | Relationship | 0 | None |

These all exhibit the same underlying form. At the top is the simple reality of the whole; on left and right are complementary finite aspects, often seen as conflicting; and at the bottom is an abstract structure which enables the finite aspects to be related. The mathematical and logical cases provide very simple examples which can help to give a sense of what is happening at the much more complex levels.

To show this another way, we can arrange the diagrams above in columns:

|  | Column 1 | Column 2 | Column 3 | Column 4 | Column 5 |
|---|---|---|---|---|---|
| Line 0: | Reality | Presence | Love | Infinity | All |
| Line 1: | Outer | Physical | Male | 1 | And |
| Line 2: | Inner | Personal | Female | $-1$ | Or |
| Line 3: | Form | Necessity | Relationship | 0 | None |

The four items in each column are related as follows:

Concepts on Line 0 evoke the quality of wholeness.

Concepts on Line 1 evoke finite common outer experience, which is externally observable. This is the natural concern of males, and is exemplified by the externality of the male sexual organs.

Column 4: we can observe 1 object

Column 5: we can observe one set AND another

set.

Concepts on Line 2 concern finite individual inner experience. It is hidden and inherently unobservable except as direct personal experience. This is the natural concern of females, and is exemplified by the internality of the female sexual organs. In Columns 4 and 5, Line 2 contains duals of Line 1 which we cannot observe externally, but which still make sense.

Column 4: we cannot observe − 1 objects

Column 5: we cannot observe one object OR another as an entity in itself.

Concepts on Line 3 are essentially null, evoking the relationships abstracted from experience. The sense of rightness which we experience in relation to mathematical and aesthetic and interpersonal truth is a recognition of form in World 3. We can talk of this experience, and in order to talk about it we can think of the form as a kind of thing. In fact however it is never separable from experience, but is the actual way in which things fit together. Metaphysically therefore it is proper to regard it as null: it is not something which we could regard as an event or object in the worlds of finite experience (Worlds 1 and 2).

## 5. ONE WORLD AND THREE

World 0 is the ground of 'isness' in which all reality subsists. There is only one unique fact which one can state about Presence: it is, it is 'out there ', it is 'here within', it is self-consistent. These four statements are statements of the one fact in terms of each of the four worlds. A few epithets point directly to World 0: one, absolute, immediate, true, unconditioned, whole, infinite, transcendent, loving, real, imaginative, creative, spirit, soul. The dimension is that in which we are aware of wholeness, worth and truth, beyond the appearances. It is implicit in all language which tries to express these realities.

The other three worlds are ultimately derivative. We can see ourselves each as a unique centre in which reality (World 0) has the opportunity of entering in a particular context in World 1, through a person whose inner experiences are facts in World 2. The relationship between events in these two worlds is shaped by necessary form (World 3) in relation to all other events. This is the ASIF parallel to the geometry of space-time in Einstein's theory.

World 1 is the domain investigated by the sciences. Their primary method is theory — experiment — revised theory, along the lines described by Sir Karl Popper. They are concerned with relationships in the physical world. They seek to identify similar situations and predict the outcome of some set of events by making the fundamental assumption of the uniformity of physical nature. This excludes World 2 by definition.

World 2 is the world of feelings, ideas, personal relationships. It is studied by psychology, psychiatry and sociology along semi-scientific lines, but there is no a priori reason why the methods of science should be particularly appropriate here. Since the experience of this world is primarily subjective it is probably a gross misconception to think it can best be approached in a similar way to physical phenomena. It is likely that while men on the whole have a deeper and more intuitive understanding of World 1, women on the whole have a deeper and more intuitive understanding of World 2.

World 3 consists of theories and structures of all kinds, including those of mathematics, art, drama, literature, music, philosophy, theology and human relationships. Mathematics seeks knowledge about World 3 by investigating the implications of axioms on the assumption that self-contradiction is not allowed. More complex theories are similarly based on the assumption of internal consistency and balance, but they are not generally as simple to express in explicit formal terms as mathematical forms, and at the ultimate level they are completely implicit.

## 6. POPPER'S WORLDS AND PLATO'S FORMS

Popper uses similar concepts. Worlds 1 and 2 as defined here are the same as his. He does not introduce World 0, which he presumably prefers to avoid discussing explicitly though it is implicit in his idea of what is real. His World 3, however, is a slightly different concept from the one outlined above. It consists of actual artefacts such as nests, spider's webs, language, libraries, books, mathematics, as well as theories and questions. In particular he is interested in the fact that libraries and other forms of stored experience constitute an objective autonomous world which exists whether or not it is used.

Popper's division is appropriate for his purposes. From the ASIF point of view, however, it is better to think of the contents of World 3 as consisting of the forms which are sensed as underlying products in Popper's World 3. On this view the concept labelled 'language', and the structures of a language, are forms in World 3, while the totality of a particular language is a set of events in Worlds 1 and 2 with a structure in World 3. In the ASIF a fact in World 3 is about an underlying structure, not about its expression in World 1 or its understanding or effect in World 2. This keeps World 3 as conceptually independent of Worlds 1 and 2 as possible.

Popper remarks on the closeness of his World 3 to Plato's forms. At first sight the contents of the ASIF World 3 may also look like them. They may be what Plato himself had at the back of his mind, but they are not what people have generally understood Plato to mean. Platonic forms are usually conceived of as eternal, and this leads to all kinds of corrupting absolutisms which have had terrible consequences in human history.

Facts in World 3 have no kind of existence in any meaningful sense until they are discovered. After they have been discovered it may feel as if they were there all the time. We can certainly say that it is *as if* this is so, but to say that they *were* there all the time is to divert attention from the primary fact that they were discovered through an act of human attention in a particular situation, and were recognized to be significant within that situation. This is the basic source of their worth and relevance.

The facts are undeniable once they are found and shown to be the necessary consequences of self-consistency or balance. What matters is their ontological status. The status we accord to facts in World 3 determines our attitude towards them — whether we regard them as having absolute power over us, or simply as representing constraints which have to be related to aspects of our experience in the other dimensions.

Whenever we talk of two objects in World 1, or two concepts in World 2, being similar, we are appealing to our immediate sense of a structure in World 3 which is common to them both. Every fact in World 3 is simply a self-consistent tautology, a null entity which confronts us with the implications of necessity / consistency — what one might call 'pure form'. The activity of discovering valuable tautologies is hard work, because it is a process of deciding which of the infinite range of possible tautologies is truly significant. It is as difficult as writing a good tune.

Once discovered, facts in World 3 are relatively easily disseminated in the form of taught knowledge, because they correspond to our immediate sense of self-consistency. This ease, however, can be a trap. Our Western way of thinking tends to devalue knowledge by ignoring the cost of achieving it: too often we see knowledge as a means of manipulation rather than a legacy to be responsibly used.

## 7. TRINITY AND DUALITY

Dimensions 1, 2 and 3 form a trinity, with a small 't', and they provide an intellectual antidote to the extremes of the scientific approach. Unless it is leavened by awareness of the subjective world scientific thinking can lead to metaphysical aridity. Much of it is based on the binary (either-or) forms found in computing, which lie at the root of logical and mathematical models of the universe. This is good when we are seeking to express things unambiguously, but the price is that it is metaphysically lifeless.

Simple logic becomes dangerously misleading when we try to generalize it to the metaphysical level. It is two-dimensional, and often traps us in a dualism involving irreconcilable conflicts in our thinking which hypnotize the mind. Dualism places opposites in confrontation with each other, presenting us with the picture of two entities which are eternally separate. Good and Evil are seen as absolutes in eternal conflict; Mind and Body contend to be treated as 'objectively real'; Life and Death are seen as struggling for 'victory'.

If we are aware of the threefoldness within reality, however, we can transform the idea of dualism into that of duality. Duality emphasizes the relationship which exists between opposites. It interprets them as complements of each other, with special strengths in different areas. It enables the imagination to explore the richness of manifold dualities. It allows us to have a clearly envisaged conception of the complex relationship between the external and internal world which frees us from any sense of the need for a 'mechanical' correspondence between the two.

The most basic form of complementarity is the relation between one and many. There are many personal universes and one physical universe; the male produces many sperm and the female one egg; presence is one and whole, while necessity is multiple but empty. The unitary self-awareness of World 0 is matched by the complex self-consistency of World 3; multiplicity in World 1 is matched by singleness in World 2, and vice versa.

Language reflects our experience intimately, and so provides innumerable examples of duality. One of the most fundamental of these is the duality between external objects and mental concepts. There are many objects to which a concept such as 'chair' applies, and there are many concepts which can be applied to the chair I am sitting on at the moment. A proposition about a particular object is an assertion that the concept behind the words properly applies to the object. Through a great number of judgments of this kind a large-scale duality is built up between objects in the world and concepts in the mind. This is how language grows and develops.

If we think in a threefold way we realize that the link between opposing entities is an essential part of the structure. Moreover, since we can form pairs in any way we choose, the mind is free to perform a continual dance as it switches the grouping from one to another of the three possible pairs. World 1 links Worlds 2 and 3 by providing a common domain in which the two can be related; World 2 links Worlds 1 and 3 to build up scientific knowledge; World 3 links Worlds 1 and 2 by providing conceptual structures which form the basis for understanding.

The threeness within the fourfold pattern can therefore be seen as more fundamental than the twofoldness of opposites. Life can be conceived of as a whole (World 0) being created out of the unendingly complex relationships between Worlds 1, 2 and 3. At every level it will exhibit the threefold pattern in innumerable ways.

## 8. THE OVERALL CONCEPTION

We can now form an overall conception (belonging to World 3) of the way things work. We can see ourselves as living at the meeting point of the three worlds, as centres of consciousness interacting with each other in a common awareness of reality. Each of us is self-awareness seeking to be itself at the point at which it experiences. To be itself, presence must be self-consistent. The null forms of self-consistency belong to World 3, and we can regard Worlds 0 and 3 as the infinite and zero poles of our experience. Between these, finite appearance is suspended, with the multiple inner worlds of persons and their single outer world in dual balance with each other. Everything (our thoughts, feelings, perceptions) is ultimately held together in World 0, unbounded wholeness.

Mathematics provides a highly simplified idea of the structure. Every infinity is in one sense the same, meaning 'bigger than any actual number we can think of', but we can define the approach to infinity as we choose. Zero indicates absence. Both infinity and zero are conceptual directions rather than values. We can choose to approach them simultaneously in such a way that the product remains finite. If y remains equal to $1/x$ as x increases (and so their logarithms balance each other arithmetically) it makes sense to say that in this case the product of infinity and zero is 1. x in World 1 and y in World 2 are held together by the mathematical relationship in World 3 which is a necessary condition that their product shall be finite. The finite '1' arises out of the relationship between x and y as they reach simultaneously towards infinity and zero.

In the human situation the details of it are complex but the heart simple. Our external and internal experiences (Worlds 1 and 2) are poised between presence and form (Worlds 0 and 3). It is intuitively clear that this means that Worlds 1 and 2 must be in balance in a metaphysical sense.

We can regard the state of our multiple internal worlds as precisely related, in terms of the necessity imposed by the forms in World 3, to the state of the physical world. The relationship is not a simple mirroring, but an infinitely complex one based on duality.

## 9. CHOICE

The question now arises, why does everything take one particular form rather than any other? The only possible answer is 'because of our choices'. Everything in the universe as described is conceptually deterministic except the way in which we live each moment: this is the only element which is ultimately variable. The basic building block of our experience is not the person but the person-moment. The one thing we know we can choose is how we as self-aware centres of consciousness relate to the truth of the present. The central choice — the only point at which pure twofoldness arises — is whether we respond YES or NO to our awareness of this truth.

The response has direct effects in practical terms, but these are merely the surface aspect. The choice which matters is deep down at the point where our root sense of the particular concrete situation tips in one direction or the other. It is beyond language, though the action of speaking or writing may be closely bound up with it. If we are in an attitude which is properly open, the way it tips will be in accordance with the real needs of the whole.

Freedom is to be found in the open attention with which we seek what is needed and the YES with which we greet it when recognized. *Between* points of decision we have to seek the course which will hold outer and inner in proper relationship and move in the direction of wholeness. *At* points of decision we are asked to assent to our true course when we recognize it. We are always at liberty to say NO if we choose to, and so to reject our own truth.

Knowledge of the 'right' direction cannot possibly be learned by instruction, because the first thing we have to decide is how to interpret the situation. We can only know it by being where we are. Awareness of it belongs to World 0, and consists in recognizing the structure in World 3 which is the true form of what is happening. YES allows wholeness to fill the relationship between Worlds 1 and 2 in a bounded volume of person-space-time. NO allows a mismatch to enter the relationship which will be reflected in the balance between World 1 and World 2. This in turn will be experienced both by ourselves and by others in the need for a new YES which represents an acceptance and transformation of the situation arising from the NO.

## 10. SIMPLE LOGIC

Undergirding root sense is the structure of personal logic which gives our sense of rightness its intellectual backbone. As a preliminary to examining personal logic we need to consider the nature of simple logic. This consists solely of the implications of non-contradiction. It is essentially null, and can be expressed completely negatively. Each of the basic logical operators (AND, OR, NOT) can be expressed in terms of the single operator 'IF ... THEN ...'. Similarly (at the next level) logical arguments are built up from statements of the form 'IF A THEN B'. This can be written in the form 'NOT (A AND NOT B)', meaning that the statements 'A IS TRUE' and 'B IS FALSE' cannot both be true.

The structure is illustrated in the diagram below. When I utter the statement 'IF A THEN B' speaking to you I appeal to our common sense of the logic shown in the table. The contents of the table show, for each combination of truth-values, whether it can actually exist:

|  |  | A IS | |
|---|---|---|---|
|  |  | TRUE | FALSE |
| B IS | ( TRUE | YES | YES |
|  | ( FALSE | NO | YES |

The whole idea of proof is built up relying on this basic conception. We accept it as a necessary condition for rational argument. Our acceptance of mathematics (to the extent that it is an understanding as opposed to a grudging acquiescence) is based on our immediate shared awareness of this structure, which is imposed by the need for non-contradiction.

Simple logic of this kind gives some feeling for the necessity imposed by form. When one comes to aesthetic and moral and personal logic, they are so much more complex and richer than mathematical logic that it is hardly surprising that they present much greater difficulties to our understanding. It is therefore to be expected that our greatest successes up ·to now have derived from mathematics and physics. They present us with relatively simple problems which even so provide taxing challenges.

The mathematical sciences have the advantage of operating in an area which we all share in common and which we have to accept as simply being there. Every insight can be tested by experiments which are agreed to be appropriate. Ironically, there is at the same time tremendous excitement in the search: it is intimately bound up with the inner drive (World 2) of the scientists and thinkers. The insights are established on the basis of an internal aesthetic sense of the way in which a whole conception of the physical universe hangs together, and this is essentially an awareness of a deep unity between our concepts and physical reality.

## 11. PERSONAL LOGIC
When we come to the fields of religion or politics or music or art it becomes much more difficult to disentangle discussion about the structure from the way it relates to reality. We are no longer able to achieve a relatively detached position, because the very fact that we are discussing them in a particular context in a particular way

forms an integral part of the argument. Nevertheless we can conceive that there are structures of consistency to be found through imaginative and open discussion, and that these structures form the basis for tackling the problems which arise.

The problems here are so complex that they call for much greater emphasis on approaches which are complementary to that of science. This is not the place to go into great detail about the ASIF view of the logic of the personal world, but I shall pick out some basic features which relate to the main argument. They point to forms which underlie the way the world is.

First, the internal world is to be seen as the dual of the external world. The exact form of the duality is determined by our choices. When Cain kills Abel, the act arises out of a choice deep inside Cain. At the metaphysical level Cain allows himself to say NO, and refuses to face up to his own pride. Instead he seeks to save it at the cost of his brother's life. His choice is reflected in a matching pair of dual distortions — a violent action in World 1, and a need to make good in World 2 which then becomes everyone's responsibility. The experienced fullness of relationship between inner and outer worlds is diminished.

Secondly, awareness is central. As we make our choices we are aware simultaneously of our whole situation — where we are, what we feel, what other people have done and would think should be done in similar situations. These are our knowledge, forming one aspect of our awareness. At the same time we are aware of our ignorance, the whole range of unknown possibilities which we cannot imagine. Our awareness is at the meeting point of these dual aspects, and seeks to recognize the direction and the moment of choice simultaneously.

The third feature concerns the nature of worth. The point of choice is the only point at which anything of real worth can happen. The deliberate costly choice of a course of action or a line of thinking is the point at which true worth enters the fabric of the universe. There is no 'merit' in making the true choice: even to think of merit is distraction from the new moment of choice. Every real human achievement arises out of the simple fact that at a particular place, at a particular time, a person recognizes the truth of the moment and responds to it. The reward consists solely in doing this.

Fourthly, at the deepest level we are completely interdependent. We are not a collection of individuals seeking our own private ends in disregard of others: we are a wholeness seeking to be itself in fathomless depth of experience. Our self-awareness is the self-awareness of the whole, and the longings we experience are the longings of self-awareness, however distorted and hampered by individual NOes, to fill the whole structure of mind, physical world and concept.

Finally, the single most important aspect of the way we live is the attitude we take to each other. If we choose to disregard the fact that each of us is a living person of equal absolute worth, even in the most apparently trivial action or thought, that moment of choice is an absolute negative which in the context of the moment shatters the fabric of the world. In this sense all our choices are moral choices. We have to grow into an attitude which continually seeks to open the way to wholeness whatever the personal cost, and whatever our personal likes and dislikes, so that it becomes the basis of all our decisions from the most minor to the greatest. This makes deep courtesy central.

The spirit of exclusiveness is totally foreign to such an attitude. Competition has its place in the world of appearances, but it has to be centred in an attitude which genuinely longs for fulfilment for all. Every human action is to be tested against the ultimate criterion — does it arise out of an integrity which seeks unconditionally to open the way to the wholeness of the whole? The crucial test for a religion is whether it is a means by which such an attitude is fostered and deepened in its adherents. Whatever its imagined authority, every religious teaching which works against such an attitude is self-condemned. At the same time there are reservoirs of strength in all religions which when purged and properly related to each other can work powerfully to dissolve the barriers between us and reality.

## 12. WORDS

Words and language have a very special relationship to our whole experience. The utterance or writing of a word is an act which links together the physical, personal and conceptual aspect of experience in a unique way. It occurs at the meeting point of outer and inner, and it is intimately bound up with the fact that it is uttered, the situation in which it is uttered, and the way in which it is uttered.

It always carries with it the implication 'this is what I choose to say now': the fact that it is uttered is a direct expression of that choice. On the other hand it does not necessarily imply the message 'this is the right thing for me to say now' or 'this is true'. We normally assume that both of these are implied, but we always have to be alert to the fact that if we take these for granted without relating properly to the speaker this in itself may be a perfectly good reason for him to 'pull our legs' — to utter a sentence which is not superficially true. The formal meaning of an expression is only one component of its whole meaning. A much more fundamental component is the implicit YES/NO which relates it to the whole context, indicating whether the expression is to be understood as true or as ironical or even deliberately false.

Words are the vehicle by which we share our experience of the truth. Part of their function is to convey simple matters of fact, and it is clear that factual inaccuracy distorts our perception of reality in matters of detail, sometimes disastrously. Much more important, however, is the total attitude conveyed by words when used with a particular tone in a particular context. A society seeking to be whole cannot evade the need for truthfulness not only of the letter but of the spirit. The newspeak indulged in by some politicians and journalists is deeply insidious and corrupting because it selects factual truth but completely distorts its significance. When the misleading use of words is justified by the need to retain power or circulation the metaphysical truth is turned upside down. The wholeness of society depends on language which conveys the reality of what is going on. The Big Lie is its enemy, destroying mutual trust and threatening the very soul of language. It is strengthened by every small lie, however apparently trivial: each temptation to collude may be a critical point in the whole struggle.

We also use words to discuss words. The capacity of words for self-transcendence is a reflection of self-awareness. If we understand this aspect of words it keeps the logical aspect in proper proportion, and throws new light on the logical paradoxes.

## 13. PARADOXES

At the turn of the century Frege and Russell were deeply disturbed by the paradox of the class of all classes which do not belong to themselves. Nowadays such paradoxes are circumvented by using axiomatic set theory or by means of a theory of types, but it is valuable to see exactly why they arise out of our natural use of language.

The source of the main paradoxes lies in the formal relationship between self-reference and negation. This will become clear if we look at one of the simplest and most elegant paradoxes, which aroused interest shortly after Russell ran into trouble.

In 1908, Kurt Grelling came up witth the heterological, or SELF-FALSE, paradox. A SELF-TRUE adjective is one whose meaning applies to itself. The negative is SELF-FALSE. Examples are:

SELF-TRUE words: one    twelve-letter    wee    English    polysyllabic

SELF-FALSE words: two    four-letter    long    French    monosyllabic

We run into the paradox when we try to decide whether the word SELF-FALSE is SELF-FALSE or SELF-TRUE. If we say 'the adjective SELF-FALSE is SELF-FALSE' we are doing two contrary things simultaneously:

saying that it belongs to the set of SELF-FALSE adjectives

demonstrating that the adjective is SELF-TRUE.

A similar thing happens if we say 'the adjective SELF-FALSE is SELF-TRUE'.

Trivial as this example may seem it pins down precisely a point which we can sense but which is extremely elusive. It is a very simple instance of the fundamental relationship between the dimensions — our self-awareness, our internal experience, our observations and our concepts.

If we have a self-referent expression, there is a conflict between the negative of the expression formed from the mental concept (the internal or subjective negative) and the negative formed from the external list of expressions. The result is that if we are to avoid self-contradiction we must split the list of adjectives into three mutually exclusive sets:

A : All SELF-TRUE adjectives including SELF-TRUE

B : All SELF-FALSE adjectives except those in C

C : The adjectives SELF-FALSE, HETEROLOGICAL
    and synonyms.

These are irreducible subsets of the English adjectives in respect of the quality SELF-TRUE. We have found an adjective which will not allow us to split the universe into two mutually exclusive sets by using negativity. The concept 'not SELF-TRUE' does not match up with the set 'not those which are SELF-TRUE'. There is a discrepancy between inner and outer worlds.

If we wish to handle the situation using simple logic, in other words to split adjectives into two mutually exclusive sets, we can certainly do so. But in order to do this we must have an agreed usage: for instance we may give the name 'unselftrue' to all adjectives which do not belong to the SELF-TRUE set, *ie.* to the set consisting of B and C. To do this we have to make a choice.

This is the heart of the matter: we are constrained by the nature of the relationship between SELF and NOT to make our own decision. Logic itself prevents us from relying entirely on logic. We have to take into account the real world and the real situations in which the words are to be used. Only these particulars can give any grounds for a decision: there is no *a priori* way in which to decide how the sets 'should' be grouped. The decision is an act of faith that in the light of all future uses it will turn out that this was the 'right' choice.

## 14. UNDERLYING PATTERNS
Further patterns underlie this example.

The concept SELF-TRUE is closely related to self-awareness. Self-awareness has a similar reflexive quality to self-truth. It involves awareness that one is aware: it is a timeless reality in which we experience consciousness. It is perhaps what Descartes really had in mind when he formulated his famous dictum *Cogito ergo sum.*

In the SELF-TRUE example there is a relationship of duality between sets B and C. There are many items in B and only one in C. We may see C as being in the position of the individual in relation to the group. There is a mutual interdependence: words in set B are a heterogeneous muddle until they are linked by the concept SELF-FALSE, while set C is a word which is of no use apart from set B, since without B it has nothing to refer to. So each needs the other, and they are united in their common relationship of negation to set A. We have in the example a simple clear-cut case of the metaphysical atom we have already discussed:

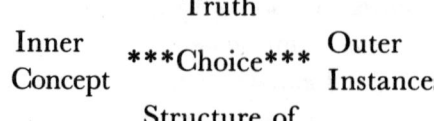

                        Truth

Inner        ***Choice***     Outer
Concept                       Instances

                   Structure of
              Self-reference & Negation

We can see the pattern of the paradox appearing in a fresh guise if we translate the picture

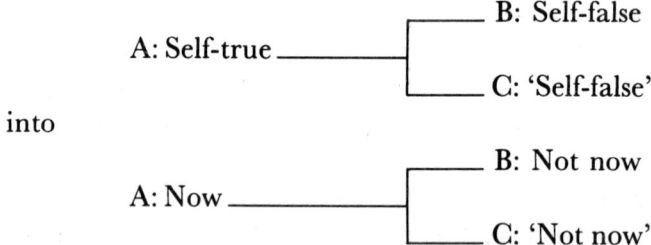

                                    ┌───── B: Self-false
          A: Self-true ─────────────┤
                                    └───── C: 'Self-false'

into

                                    ┌───── B: Not now
          A: Now ───────────────────┤
                                    └───── C: 'Not now'

Here B (Not now) is the past or the future viewed as a collection of physical facts. C ('Not now') is the past or future viewed as a concept or hypothesis. Our life is a continuous search to hold the two apparently irreconcilable aspects together. This can only be done by an act of imagination which continually seeks to integrate the multiplicity of B with the singleness of C.

We have used logic itself to show that at the very core of logic choice enters as an ineradicable element. In Mathematics this leads to Gödel's theorem. In computing it means that a system can never be proved correct without going outside the system. In business it means that however carefully rules are laid down situations always arise which require a decision on the unique case. In morals it means that while in the bulk of cases a particular defined pattern of action is usually the right one it is never an automatic thing, and there are always individual cases where one must transcend the norms.

We can extend this argument to the widest context. 'Not now' refers both forwards to the future and backwards to the past. Past and future are like right and left and are closely related to them: we have an absolute sense of their 'direction' which we cannot escape, and this is built into our minds and our bodies. But our self-awareness stands above and beyond past and future: it is simply a 'now' in which our conceptions of the past and future are related.

Once we break free of the idea that facts in Worlds 1, 2 or 3 (whether in the past or the future) are absolute, we can recognize that it is not they which are primary, but the rightness of the relationship between them. This rightness resides in self-awareness which takes into account the whole state of the cosmos at each moment and transforms it precisely in accordance with the choices that are made. Worlds 1, 2 and 3 become the ways in which self-awareness beyond experience presents the truth of the whole to self-awareness within each person.

The concept also frees us from the need to postulate a beginning or end for the physical universe. Although our experience of ordinary life suggests that there must be a beginning and an end, we forget that such an analogy is anthropocentric, inferred from the finiteness of our lives. Self-awareness lies in a dimension which contains and transcends finiteness. The past is continuously created just as the future is continuously created, and beginnings and ends are simply meaningless at the ultimate metaphysical level.

None of this contradicts commonsense notions of physical and personal facts. It simply introduces a shift of perspective which parallels the shift of perspective provided by the Theory of Relativity. Relativity sees the way in which the universe develops as directly related to the current and past configuration of matter. The ASIF sees each moment as a precise fleshing out of the whole pattern of individual choices. It interprets the whole present situation of each one of us, every aspect of it, as the presentation in our own personal language of the state of the whole as it stands at the moment.

## 15. CREATION MODELS

This is an overwhelming concept if we try to work out its implications in an exhaustive way. Its value is as a theoretical construct which protects us from illusions and logical traps when we try to form a conception of the working of the whole. As an illustration of its use, we can consider models of creation.

We can examine three main models: the Biblical story of the Creation and Fall, the evolutionary idea of gradual development, and the Hindu idea of an eternal cycle. Each has its weaknesses. The Biblical story is always in danger of suggesting a God who is outside creation, and has no satisfactory explanation of the existence of evil, which it seems must have been ultimately created by God. The evolutionary model can give rise to the unsatisfactory notion of endless progress, and this can undermine any sense of the need for costly moral choice. The Hindu version is liable to lead to a fatalistic sense of endless recurrence. Each view can easily trap us in a finite vision based on a two-dimensional picture.

The ASIF suggests something more along the lines of a 'random walk'. In our own experience we know there are times when there are opportunities we miss or errors we make through simple failure to trust our own judgment. These are choices for which we alone have the responsibility: we are free to respond YES or NO. YES calls for trust in our root sense beyond the appearances. It can be hard, but it pins the structure of creation to reality at that point. NO is a rupture which sends a judder through the whole system.

When we think of creation we can therefore picture it as a response to the YESes and NOes as they have actually been made. Theoretically it would be possible for all the choices to have been YESes. In practice it has turned out that they are a complete mixture. What we have is a world which is precisely appropriate to that pattern of choices.

But the 'walk' is not in fact truly random. If it were it would be much the same as the cyclical conception, continuing arbitrarily for ever. This would suggest that we are completely imprisoned, and would close off the openness which lies at the heart of a true conception. Each choice is made not at random but as a deliberate decision. NO blocks the way for everyone, while YES opens the way to endless possibility. When we wake up to this and assent to it the randomness is transformed into creativity.

Even the idea of a 'walk' is not wholly satisfactory. It still contains the idea of travelling through clock time, and clock time is itself part of the conceptual structure through which we relate to each other and to our experience. We come closer to an adequate conception if we think of the whole universe not as progressing in time but as a complex structure of matching events in Worlds 1 and 2 which grows in richness and depth around and within the eternal present moment.

It is conceivable that a state can be reached in which the YESes take off so that the whole is caught up into a kind of metadimension. This is the conception underlying ideas of Utopia and the Second Coming. However, any attempt to derive consolation from such a possibility would be a distraction. The value of such an idea is essentially negative: it prevents us from closing off our thinking (and thereby distorting our emotional response) by assuming that ultimate fulfilment is impossible. As far as our understanding and attitude are concerned its status is undecidable — we should treat it as neither possible nor impossible, in the category of a dream which may or may not be related to reality. We can legitimately be determined that it shall be possible, but we must not treat it as in any sense a foregone conclusion, or link it inextricably with any specific image or temporal prediction.

## 16. A LINGUISTIC DISTINCTION

The fourfold pattern forms a cross. This suggests a basic distinction which can be valuable when analysing our use of language. The vertical elements (0 and 3) have the primary quality of infinity, while the horizontal elements (1 and 2) have the primary quality of finiteness. Worth resides solely in the vertical elements, and relationship in the horizontal. This is closely akin to the common distinction between value and fact. Any sentence may contain both elements explicitly. The context and the way in which the sentence is uttered also carry implicit overtones.

A command conveys the implication 'this is what you must do'. It contains a hidden appeal to the rightness reqired by the whole state of affairs. R.M. Hare in *The Language of Morals* calls this the 'neustic' element — the 'nod of the head' — in the command. It belongs to Dimension 0, the dimension of self-awareness and worth. It relies on the authority implicit in the requirements of the present moment. There is a pure 'ought' (independent of any individual or social authority's expressed prescription) which underlies this component of language.

The neustic element is present in scientific language in a subtle way. When a scientist announces that the creation of the world took place in a Big Bang he implies that because of his status and integrity, backed up by the status and integrity of the vast army of scientists, we 'ought' to accept what he says, and take it that this is what 'really' happened. Our mental conditioning makes it hard to free ourselves of the idea that first there 'was' the Big Bang, and then the galaxies 'came into being' and life 'began', and so on, and that these are the 'real' facts which happened objectively in sequence. Reality lies in the vertical dimension: relationship within time lies in the horizontal. The theories simply tell us that to the best of our knowledge everything now is related *as if* this theory is correct. We are too easily led to metaphysical conclusions which are not justified. The fact that in the model the Big Bang precedes choice in clock time does not entail that it is metaphysically prior.

Similar confusions surround the question of the existence of God. The word 'God' is an extremely powerful word because of what it has meant and means in the lives of men and women. It is associated with ways of thinking about the whole which have profound effects on our conduct and on our relations with each other. It is a symbol for World o — Reality — while 'existence' is normally used as a symbol for continuity in time in the finite worlds. 'God exists' is therefore a statement containing a grammatical confusion unless we interpret 'exists' as 'is real'. The statement then becomes 'Reality is real', with which it is hard to disagree.

As individuals we have a simple choice in respect of the experience which some people call 'belief in God'. It is a naked experience of the vertical dimension, not an intellectual thing, in which we choose to trust or deny what we are aware of as the real truth where we are. However the public use of the word God must depend on circumstances, because its abuse throughout history has on occasions made it necessary to rebel against it. Verbally denying the existence of God can even be an act of trust in God in some circumstances. When the word is not a weapon in the power struggle, however, it can be a symbol for World o, just as at the other end of the metaphysical spectrum 'o' is the symbol for absolute emptiness.

The phrase 'life after death' is another example of verbal confusion. It is a metaphorical way of speaking which nowadays is not very helpful unless people can see through the literal meaning. The word 'after' belongs to the finite world, while the word 'life' as used here belongs to the vertical world, the world of the soul. The words are an attempt to express the sense that presence transcends and contains every event in the other worlds. To translate this into words involving clock time is not possible.

In these examples we have been identifying the finite and infinite elements. We are making the familiar distinction between fact and value/worth. Facts in Worlds 1 and 2 lie in the horizontal realm. Worth lies in the vertical realm, and it is fleshed out as Worlds 1 and 2 are related to each other and to the whole in the context of World 3. Our use of words is a major element of this fleshing out, and the metaphysical distinction between vertical and horizontal realms (uncreated/created, real/relational) must be respected whenever we speak or write.

In particular the ancient philosophical chestnut 'Can one get an ought from an is?' can be seen as another attempt to confuse ourselves — or as an examination question to test whether we can see through the confusion. Metaphysically 'ought' belongs to the vertical realm and 'is' to the horizontal realm, and so they are formally independent. However, in reality they are precisely linked at every point of decision. The answer to the question is a simultaneous 'Never' and 'Always', each being understood in its appropriate dimension.

## 17. MEETNESS

In speaking of right choice we can talk of it as 'appropriate to the circumstances'. However 'appropriateness' is not usually a strong word: it tends to suggest good form, conformity with an established pattern. Taken in this sense it is the exact opposite of what is required: it omits the elements of newness and uniqueness which are essential to what is happening.

In a strong sense, however, appropriateness is the expression of worth. It requires a fitting match between context, thought and action. The old English word 'meet' expresses it with characteristic four-letter vigour, and it is sad and perhaps significant that it has virtually disappeared from our vocabulary. Our current adjectives 'fitting', 'apt', 'proper', 'suitable' are poor relatives. They have lost the simple strength of the idea that at any moment there is a single way which is meet for the unique situation.

Meetness lies close to the heart of this country's best values — fairness, consideration, gentlemanliness, respect, team spirit, courtesy, sportsmanship, the proper thing. These terms are easily mocked. They have become tarnished through being confined to particular groups in society, so denying the comprehensiveness which is essential to them. They are values without bounds, since they must always be open to fresh circumstances, and are based on an idea of worth which takes everyone and everything in the situation into full account.

## 18. PRACTICAL IMPLICATIONS

There are many practical implications of the ASIF, and I here pick out a handful.

One implication is very simple. Whatever our feelings and knowledge and circumstances, they are a plain statement to us of the state of the whole. Everything we experience as disharmony and offence and pain is a legacy of choices which have been shirked. We live in a universe which we must treat as closed backwards and open forwards. We have to seek a proper relationship between the closed past and the open future by interpreting each message from our circumstances and finding what it implies.

A second implication concerns the nature of decision-making. We are linked with each other through World 1.

This requires continual decisions, and most fundamental of all is recognition of the point at which a decision has to be taken. We can only sense this by being aware of the relationship between the moment and the whole. One of the hardest such tests is to recognize that we have followed a course long enough and have reached a turning point. It is frequently too hard for those in positions of power, with tragic consequences. Decisions can never be separated from time: they often take the form of choosing between the old and the new, and the question is not 'which is right in itself?', but 'which is right now in these circumstances?'

A further implication is the true nature of equality. We are each unique, with our own position in the scheme of things, and so any politically defined notion of equality is bound to be ultimately inadequate. This is not to say that the attempt to achieve it is worthless. Our real equality lies in the fact that we are all in the same metaphysical position: we are each responsible for enabling presence to fill the point where we are, and each YES is of equal absolute worth. The Biblical stories of the widow's mite and the labourers in the vineyard bring this home in vivid terms.

Moreover, since we are metaphysically a single whole, we have to accept responsibility for every NO: we have to treat it as if it is our own fault. It lies in the past once it has happened, and it presents us with a cost in some form in the present. However, each YES is a living thing, while each NO is dead: a vast number of NOes can be balanced by a single YES.

A fifth implication is that the existence of a person means that he or she is a necessary part of the whole situation. Any attempt to deny the reality of a person by the use of force in however subtle a form is futile self-deception which only increases the problem. People who disagree with us are in a position to contribute something which is beyond our own powers. We can argue with and oppose each other as much as we need to so long as we do not disregard and ride rough-shod over the eternal underlying wholeness which each of us is. True disagreements arise because people have complementary viewpoints. They can only be resolved properly when we recognize that they arise out of the relationships that lie between us and not as a result of an imagined eternal irreconcilability. That is, as has been suggested by earlier arguments, a self-contradictory notion, however difficult it may be to acknowledge.

At the same time people may cut themselves off, for the time being at least, from the truth of the situation, and others may see that this has happened. In such cases every positive method of handling the position must be regarded as admissible, provided it is based on a true assessment and provided it respects individual freedom. Any solution must seek to link to the self-awareness in the other person in a joint struggle with the root of his intransigence. What is clearly recognized as evil has to be treated as absolutely real as long as it exists, right up to the point where it is embraced by self-awareness. But it must never be seen as inextricably linked with the living person.

There is a great list of further implications, but I will mention only one more here. It concerns the whole approach to education. The most important thing for a child to learn from the very start is that he is not practising for life but is actually living in the present. This is not to expect a suddenly adult sense of responsibility, but simply to encourage by every means the sense that the child has a unique part to play, equally with his peers and with his elders, in being fully himself at every stage of life. It can only come about if the child senses that those around really believe this, and if he recognizes that others have needs of equal status to his own.

These are all ideas to which many people would assent. The ASIF may point towards a conceptual basis for realizing that they are not to be seen as some ideal (but by inference unattainable) way, but as the necessary and only way which is always there to be found.

## 19. NOW

We find ourselves at the present moment with a particular choice pattern already established. We experience our particular presentation of external and internal and conceptual worlds, with all its disharmonies and sufferings. We can conceive of these as being generated in an incommensurably dual way from the YES/NOes. The whole structure remains self-consistent in relation to what has been, what is and what is to come: it floats in the boundless sea of present reality.

Every YES has the sole worth of 'for its own sake' and of 'being oneself', and fills out the structure of the universe in the region of the moment in which it occurs. What can happen if the filling out reaches a level at which it becomes self-generating is beyond our powers of imagination. It is matched in deadly seriousness by its physical dual — the self-generation of the atomic bomb.

Everything depends on individual integrity trusting and expressing the integrity of the whole within each particular context. What matters is that we continually open ourselves with deliberate intent to the needs of the endlessly differentiated whole as we encounter it in each real situation. While this necessarily entails personal cost and suffering, and sometimes feelings of hopelessness and despair, no degree of sophistication can undermine the intellectual coherence of such an attitude and the worth of living it out in full.

# ACKNOWLEDGEMENTS

The list below acknowledges the sources of quotations and other books referred to either directly or indirectly.

Barrett, William
*The Illusion of Technique* (Kimber)
Bede, The Venerable
*A History of the English Church and People* (Penguin)
Berkeley, G.
*Three Dialogues* (Open Court, Illinois)
Capra, Fritjof
*The Turning Point* (Flamingo)
Dawkins, Richard
*The Extended Phenotype* (OUP)
*The Blind Watchmaker* (Longman)
*The Selfish Gene* (OUP)
Eliot, T.S.
*Four Quartets* (Faber & Faber)
*Murder in the Cathedral* (Faber & Faber)
*Encyclopedia of Ignorance* (Pergamon)
*Encyclopedia of Philosophy* (Macmillan)
*English Hymnal* (OUP)
*Fontana Dictionary of Modern Thought* (Collins)
Hare, R.M.
*The Language of Morals* (OUP)
Hawking, Stephen
*A Brief History of Time* (Bantam)

Kierkegaard, S.A.
  *The Last Years* (Ed. & Tr. R. Gregor Smith) (Collins)
Le Corbusier
  *The Modulor* (Faber)
Magee, Bryan
  *Men of Ideas* (BBC)
  *Modern British Philosophy* (OUP)
  *Popper* (Fontana)
  *Schopenhauer* (OUP)
Phillips, J.B.
  *Your God is too small* (Epworth)
Plato
  *Republic* (Tr. Lee) (Penguin)
Popper, Karl
  *Conjectures and Refutations* (Routledge and Kegan Paul)
  *Objective Knowledge* (OUP)
  *The Open Society and Its Enemies* (Routledge and Kegan Paul)
  *Unended Quest* (Fontana)
Wittgenstein, Ludwig
  *Tractatus Logico-Philosophicus* (Routledge and Kegan Paul)
  *Philosophical Investigations* (Basil Blackwell)
Yourcenar, M.
  *Memoirs of Hadrian* (Plon)
Zaehner, R.C.
  *The Concise Encyclopedia of Living Faiths* (Hutchinson)

# APPENDIX A: THE PROOF OF THREENESS

The 'self-false paradox' arises when we consider the set of all adjectives which refer (apply) to themselves. Such adjectives are called 'self-true', and examples are 'English', 'wee' and 'one'. There is no problem with most such adjectives: it is normally quite clear whether they are self-true or self-false, and even if we are uncertain the decision is simply a practical problem of interpreting the meaning.

However, one adjective presents us with a logical paradox. Kurt Grelling called attention to it in 1908 (he called the self-true adjectives 'autological', and the self-false 'heterological'). The problem arises with the adjective which means 'not self-true', viz. 'self-false'. If this refers to itself it is self-true, which by its own definition it is not. If it does not refer to itself it is self-false, and therefore it applies to itself. So there is a paradox — it cannot be either self-true or self-false.

We therefore need to partition adjectives not into two but into three sets, which we can display as follows:

| Self-true | Not self-true |
|---|---|
| All self-true adjectives including 'self-true' | The adjective 'self-false' |
| | Adjectives other than 'self-false' which do not refer to themselves. |

The two sets on the right together form the total of words

which are not self-true. We are forced to split them because not to do so results in a contradiction.

This example shows that when self-reference is involved it is necessary to have at least three fundamental sets, and not two as is assumed by logic. The system of categories appropriate for external items (in this case words) cannot be a binary system in respect of a reflexive attribute.

We can now state a general theorem arising out of the paradoxes of self-reference. We can define a self-referent category as a category (of expressions) whose members belong to the set to which they refer. Then the following theorem can be stated.

The Self-true Theorem:
  A self-referent category splits the universe of discourse into three irreducible sets.

Proof:
If the expression for the category is 'A', it consists of a totality of members A, and by the definition of 'A' each member of A belongs to the set to which it refers.

Suppose that there is single category 'B' which points to all the members of the universe which do not belong to A. Then its members (applying 'not' to the definition of 'A') do not belong to the class to which they refer. The totality of these members is B, and by the definition of 'B' each member of B does not belong to the set to which it refers.

Then if the expression 'B' belongs to B it does not belong to itself (by the definition of 'B'). This is a contradiction and so the expression cannot belong to B.

Also if the expression 'B' belongs to A, it belongs to itself (by the definition of 'A') and so it is a member of B. But if it is a member of B it does not belong to itself. This is a contradiction and so the expression cannot belong to A.

The hypothesis that there is a single category 'B' which points to a single totality B is therefore false. Since the minimum number of categories above one is two, we conclude that the most basic legitimate division of the universe of discourse is into the three sets:

1.  A          (including 'A')
2.  'B'                              (or 'not A')
3.  B          (excluding 'B')       (or not A)

The expression for the negative category forms a set on its own, and the assumption that we can always split reality into two mutually exclusive sets is shown to be false.

This constitutes the Proof of Threeness. It shows that in the last resort reality can never be completely reduced to pairs of mutually exclusive sets. If we wish to split the entities into two physical sets on the basis of self-referent categories, *someone* has to make a decision about the name 'not A' — *it cannot be automatic.*

This argument applies to the 'class of all classes' paradox and to the 'all generalizations are false' paradox — in fact to any paradox which is based on self-reference. It arises out of the inherent relationship between self-reference and negativity / love and logic / life and death.

# APPENDIX B: TRINITIES AND DUALITIES

There is an endless list of trinities which exhibit the kind of threefoldness which is discussed in Chapter 6. The list below will help to give some idea of the concept but is in no way definitive. The choice of order is generally arbitrary and I have not attempted to impose any formal regularity. There is also a good deal of overlapping: the concept is very fluid, since every pair can be linked by a great range of third members. There is no 'right' trinity except for the particular situation.

| | | | |
|---|---|---|---|
| Action | Attitude | Vision | |
| Action | Manner | Word | |
| Action | Method | Goal | |
| Active | Passive | Middle | (Greek tenses) |
| African | European | Asian | |
| Artisan | Bourgeois | Intelligentsia | |
| Athlete | Artist | Thinker | |
| Balanced | Biased | Woolly | |
| Brahma | Vishnu | Siva | |
| Brave | Foolhardy | Frightened | |
| Buddhism | Christianity | Islam | |
| Coherent | Incoherent | Pedantic | |
| Concealment | Flaunting | Honesty | |
| Conservative | Socialist | Liberal | |
| Craftsman | Engineer | Scientist | |
| Creation | Destruction | Conservation | |

| | | | |
|---|---|---|---|
| Creation | Person | Truth | |
| Decision | Action | Criticism | |
| Determinism | Freedom | Attitude | |
| Drive | Relaxation | Sensitivity | |
| Earth | Heaven | Human life | |
| Enthusiasm | Caution | Judgment | |
| Exaggerate | Play down | Describe | |
| Extravagant | Mean | Measured | |
| Faith | Hope | Charity | |
| Father | Son | Holy Spirit | |
| Feeling | Thinking | Willing | |
| Finite | Zero | Infinite | |
| French | German | English | |
| Future | Past | Present | |
| Giver | Acceptor | Gift | |
| God | Freedom | Immortality | (Kant) |
| Greek | Jewish | Christian | |
| Hinduism | Buddhism | Jainism | (India) |
| Honest | Casual | Dishonest | |
| Individual | Social | Creative | |
| Intention | Determination | Execution | |
| Judaism | Christianity | Islam | |
| Land | Water | Air | |
| Logic | Love | Truuth | |
| Love | Creation | Choice | |
| Male | Female | Child | |
| Masculine | Feminine | Neuter | |
| Mathematical | Aesthetic | Spiritual | |
| Mind | Body | Word | |
| One | Two | Three | |
| Open | Dogmatic | Critical | |
| Optimism | Pessimism | Hope | |
| Orthodox | Catholic | Reformed | |
| Particular | General | Actual | |
| Passive | Active | Unitive | |

| | | | |
|---|---|---|---|
| Past | Present | Future | |
| Perfect | Ideal | Distorted | |
| Physical | Biological | Personal | |
| Physical | Personal | True | |
| Physics | Biology | Psychology | |
| Pleasure | Pain | Acceptance | |
| Positive | Balanced | Negative | |
| Prayer | Work | War | (Medieval triad) |
| Prayer | Work | Peace | (New triad?) |
| Quantity | Quality | Unity | |
| Rational | Mature | Irrational | |
| Red | Green | Blue | |
| Seeing | Feeling | Hearing | |
| Semitic | Aryan | Oriental | |
| Sensory | Affective | Conceptual | |
| Sport | Art | Learning | |
| Static | Dynamic | Balanced | |
| Strong | Weak | Responsible | |
| Subject | Object | Consciousness | |
| Thesis | Antithesis | Union | |
| Thinking | Desiring | Doing | |
| Thought | Decision | Action | |
| Thought | Word | Deed | |
| Tolerant | Intolerant | Ignorant | |
| Tonic | Dominant | Subdominant | |
| True | False | Unknown | |
| Unified | Parochial | Disorganized | |
| Verbal | Visual | Intentional | |
| What | How | Why | |
| Whole | Partial | Isolated | |
| World | Flesh | Devil | |

Dualities arise out of trinities in all kinds of ways. Several examples were give in Chapter 7. Here is a longer list:

| | | |
|---|---|---|
| adjective/noun | industry/arts | position/velocity |
| adversarial/consensual | infinite/finite | positive/negative |
| all/none | inner/outer | presence/absence |
| and/or | input/output | public/private |
| Apollonian/Dionysian | knowledge/ignorance | quality/quantity |
| believer/atheist | known/unknown | rational/irrational |
| class/member | land/sea | real/imaginary |
| concept/object | left/right | rest/change |
| container/content | life/death | same/different |
| cube/sphere | light/darkness | science/religion |
| culture/society | line/point | seek/see |
| Darwinian/Lamarckian | lingam/yoni | something/nothing |
| fixed/variable | longitude/latitude | square/circle |
| form/content | love/logic | subject/object |
| full/empty | male/female | theory/practice |
| general/particular | mental/physical | things/people |
| handmade/mass-produced | mind/body | this/those |
| Heaven/Hell | noun/verb | time/space |
| hierarchical/egalitarian | now/then | top-down/bottom-up |
| hot/cold | objective/subjective | United Kingdom/Continent |
| idea/event | old/new | vertical/horizontal |
| idea/fact | one/many | war/peace |
| idealist/realist | optimism/pessimism | wife/mistress |
| immanent/transcendent | past/future | yes/no |
| individual/community | physical/personal | yin/yang |

# APPENDIX C: SEEDS

The thoughts below were among those jotted down while writing the book, but are not in it explicitly. They are not intended to be read through solidly, but if taken in small doses they may add a bit of background to the book and spark off further ideas.

We generally work outwards from what we can see to what is not seen. It is sometimes better to work the other way round.

Understanding should not demystify: it should increase our sense of wonder.

We too easily think of knowledge as power, to be used for manipulation. Knowledge has been gained at a cost, and if we do not respect it it will bring that fact home to us sooner or later.

A hypercritical attitude is the wrong approach for the deep truths — one is seeking insight, not proof.

Mental objects are as 'real' as physical objects — no more and no less.

Truth / rightness is not a category. It is neither definable nor undefinable, but a living reality.

The proper general goal is not happiness but fulfilment.

Silence directs our attention to the reality beyond and within the words. We have to speak so that others hear the silence, and listen so that we do.

'Render unto Caesar . . .' is brilliant, because *we* have to decide which is which.

'Love your neighbour as yourself' (Mark 12:31): 'as' can be understood in the sense of 'as being'.

Christ teaches us to trust beyond the darkness, but the darkness is still dark.

Christ offers true Gnosis. The Gnostics kept their knowledge secret because they feared its abuse. Christ reveals a knowledge which transcends such fear, because it is available to everyone and is beyond the possibility of ultimate abuse.

Jesus's fulfilment of the prophecies is not an automatic or mechanical thing, but an example of the way in which past, present and future are made one when presence is fully present.

Will = determination (ironically!). It is not the poor blind force envisaged by Schopenhauer, but a totally self-aware intention.

The will revealed in war is astonishing. But it is nothing compared with pure will, which is a calm determination that all shall be well.

The message of words may be in the sense, or the feel, or both.

Things are messages from the past.

If I know something and you know the same thing, there is redundancy. We need complementary knowledge just as much as common knowledge.

Money represents necessity: that is why it always tends away from balance. Balance can only be maintained by awareness, by life.

Openness of information depends on trust. It may not be right to give information if you *know* it is going to be used wrongly.

The nature of a space depends on the quality of the people sharing it. The space around the disciples and Jesus after the resurrection was a transfigured space.

We can still think of the inner world as one even though it is 'split up' between all of humanity.

No one can draw as straight a line without a good ruler as with. We have to use technology whenever it is available and right for the job.

A word encapsulates not an object but a situation (the set of relationships within which the object 'exists'). It always includes the meta-level by implication.

Moral condemnation can be a form of force, making people act out of fear.

What matters is not only the action, but the message that it conveys.

Treating zero as a special case (or as an error) is dualistic. It took genius to see zero as a member of the set of integers.

Statistics are based on the assumption that normal care is exercised. They can never be an excuse for lack of care.

Guilt is often the result of wrong ideas. We are not guilty for what we did not permit or intend. But we *are* responsible for making it good in any way we can.

We inherit a mess which is our responsibility.

The point of discipline is not to earn the right to a reward: it is to provide a framework in which real work can be done.

There are normally two primary orthogonal models for every situation, and we have to discover the model which transcends them both.

Great tragedy gives you the sense that despite the outcome the suffering was necessary and ultimately meaningful, even though the meaning cannot be expressed directly. It is expressed solely in the play.

We can usually say what the ideal would be if we were starting from scratch. Then we have to recognize that we are starting from where we are, and that the 'ideal' may actually be wrong.

The principle of stories which teach that 'good' wins in the end is right in implying that the world is a moral world, but wrong if it suggests automatic victory.

Any religious or spiritual or intellectual discipline is to be judged by whether it works towards wholeness in the individuals practising it.

Reality *is* faith.

The more meaningless the more potentially worthwhile.

There is no arbitrariness in root-sense knowledge: it is precisely related to everything in the moment.

The stance in Tai Chi epitomizes the mental stance we should have — slightly bent so that we are firmly based but not rigid.

Justice hasn't time to wait for the law.

'Beyond Good and Evil' suggests that they should be dispensed with and left behind. In fact they should be transcended — an entirely different notion.

Living on one's own gives a taste of the life of the whole — everything is interdependent. Each mistake costs double: you lose the time and you also have to correct the mistake.

There must be some critical level of awareness at which space-time itself is transformed — like the atomic bomb's critical mass.

What stops us moving mountains is the belief that it is impossible.

If after trying everything you 'fail' it is a sign that the world has not yet reached the stage where success is possible. The failure can still be absorbed into yourself.

The difference between Stoic and Christian is the latter's quiet determination that suffering can be transformed.

You can never talk about pain in general — it is always particular.

Our freedom arises because each of us is where he/she is and has to choose how to be there.

Surprise is essential. So is humour.

Right / left is a physical constant, like the direction of time. Things must be put into boxes to make communicable sense. But to understand one must understand the limitations of the boxes.

When threatened by the horns of the dilemma you take hold of them with your imagination and leap over them — like the Cretan dancers.

Everything created has a cost.

Any hint of compulsion becomes part of the negative fabric of the world.

We are all seeking the same integrity from different viewpoints.

It is willingness to do everything possible which reconciles.

The miracle only happens if you've done all you can.

We know little of the origins of many of the institutions and creations (*eg.* music). Why should we know much about the origin of everything?

Our attitude determines the properties of the space around us.

We each have to be equally aware of what is needed here and now. Religion is nothing if it distracts from this.

Everyone says that decision-making is crucial, and at the same time few recognize that it is an entirely spiritual activity.

What is right depends on the stage we are all at.

Logical circularity is stopped by the interdependence of particular and general.

An action is also a message.

'As it is in heaven': heaven is awareness of the potential, but the potential must be realized in the earth by the reality of our choices.

Our opinion matters simply because we have it, and for that reason it should be expressed appropriately. But if it does not prevail and if the decision is honestly arrived at we must accept the fact. It is still ours, because we have contributed all we could to it.

The worth of a discussion lies in the honesty with which it is pursued.

The mini-roundabout is a symbol of the true way. It provides a notional centre around which traffic can interact with mutual consideration and advantage. The alternatives (STOP signs and traffic lights) are more wasteful, potentially dangerous and authoritarian.

Renaissance Man is an obsolete ideal.

Reason destroyed the old illusions and replaced them with new ones.

'Sorry, mate'. There is a recognition of common humanity in the 'mate', but also the callousness of 'You're on your own and it's no business of mine'.

No one can properly be completely prescriptive for someone else — only analytic and descriptive and supportive.

English, having two bases (Anglo-Saxon and Latin/Greek, Plebeian and Aristocratic) for many words, embodies the idea of complementarity at its heart.

True religion is whatever makes for wholeness.

Factual knowledge and education enable us to avoid the gross mistakes. Only inner knowledge enables us to grow fully into where we are.

The fact that we often find 'goodness' boring is itself a reflection of our condition.

We all share aloneness.

A symbol without an understood context is meaningless; with one, it can be quite precise.

The aim of art is not to imitate life but to breathe the magic of life into ever fresh forms.

The world is being continuously rearranged around the present moment. The rearrangement is subject to conditions involving the relationship between time and space, and so ideas have to have time to grow into the material world.

# APPENDIX D: THE COMPLETE TRIANGLE

Since ancient times the geometry of the triangle has been recognized as one of the most beautifully simple fields of mathematical study. The reflections which follow point to the way in which it links up with some of the ideas in Part II. A basic knowledge of elementary mathematics is all that is assumed.

## 1. PYTHAGORAS AND THREEFOLDNESS

Pythagoras's theorem reveals a threefold pattern of self-reference. By dropping a perpendicular from the right-angled vertex to the hypotenuse we can divide it into two smaller triangles, and each of these triangles is similar to the whole triangle. The sub-triangles and the whole triangle all have the same shape: they are linked by the abstract idea of a triangle with a particular angle (though it is worth noticing that the outer triangle is the opposite way round to the others and so cannot be 'fitted' to the others unless it is turned over in a third dimension).

This leads to one of the best intuitive proofs of Pythagoras's theorem. Suppose that the sides enclosing the right angle have lengths a and b, and the hypotenuse has length c. Because the triangles are similar, one part of the hypotenuse has length a * (a/c) and the other has length b * (b/c). So c is made up of these two proportional parts, *ie*:

$$c = a * (a/c) + b * (b/c)$$

Multiplying both sides by c, we have:

$$c * c = a * a + b * b$$

which is Pythagoras's Theorem.

The theorem illustrates very simply the relationship between Worlds 1, 2 and 3. The lengths a and b, though superficially independent (being at right angles to each other) are linked to each other through the relationship to the hypotenuse which is expressed in the theorem. For each particular value of c, there is an infinite set of pairs a and b which are in a precisely defined dual relationship to each other. The relationship arises out of the intrinsic proportionality within the triangle.

## 2. THE 'IDEAL' RIGHT-ANGLED TRIANGLE

In the spirit of the Ancient Greeks we may look for the 'ideal' right-angled triangle. One candidate is the isosceles triangle in which the angles are 45 degrees. This is a rather dull ideal, resembling pure egalitarianism. Similarly a triangle of 30 and 60 degrees has a kind of perfection. One side is related to the hypotenuse in the ratio 1:2, and if you put two such triangles together you have an equilateral triangle. But this is still limited and rather dull. These are in a sense two extremes of the idea of an 'ideal' right-angled triangle. They are essentially static, like Plato's forms, and will be ignored in what follows.

There is a much more interesting candidate lying between these two: the triangle in which the areas of the triangles formed by dropping the perpendicular are related in the proportion of the Golden Mean. The ancients were rightly fascinated by this proportion: it symbolizes and embodies the perfect relationship between inner and outer. If we have a line LN

M

L _____ N

< ------------ I ------------ >

< --- g ---- > <---- h ---- >

whose length is 1 metre, then the Golden Mean LM is the
length which divides LN in such a way that the ratio of h
to g is the same as the ratio of g to the whole length: the
internal and external ratios are in harmony. If we work out
what this means we see that h = g * g (since the ratio of g
to 1 is g). So g and h together add to 1, *ie.*

$$g + g*g = 1$$

The solution to this equation is the Golden Mean

$$g = 0.61803...,$$

*ie.* the length of LM is approximately 618.03 millimetres.

Using this length we can form a right-angled triangle in
which there is complete internal and external harmony: the
sides and the perpendicular are in the proportions 1 :r : r*r
: r*r*r, where

$$r = \text{square root of } g = 0.78615... \ .$$

We can continue dividing up the smaller triangles indefinitely, and the sides of each triangle will be related to those
of the next larger by a factor r.

This triangle therefore provides an endless integrated
succession of dual triangles. Rather than call it 'ideal' it
seems better to emphasize the rich complementarity by
calling it the Complete Triangle.

Before discussing the properties of the triangle further, we
can see how it can be constructed out of two squares and
three circles. Instead of attempting the ancient but
impossible ideal of 'squaring the circle', we combine squares
and circles so that they generate a perfect relationship
which symbolizes the proper relationship between male and
female. The construction is reminiscent of Le Corbusier's
Modulor.

## 3. CONSTRUCTING THE COMPLETE TRIANGLE

The construction is used (sideways) on the dust wrapper of this volume. The formal description is as follows:

Construct two squares side by side, with the right side of one forming the left side of the other. Label the corners ABPQ, starting at the bottom left-hand corner and reading anti-clockwise. Call the length of the bottom line 1 unit, so that AB and QP are 1 unit long, and BP and QA are ½ unit long.

Construct Circle 1 with the top right-hand corner P as centre and with radius ½ unit.

Construct Circle 2 with the bottom left-hand corner A as centre so that it touches Circle 1 at the point in the right-hand square where AP meets Circle 1. The radius of this circle is the Golden Mean g.

Construct Circle 3 with AB as diameter. Give the label C to the point where Circle 3 meets Circle 2 in the left-hand square. Then ABC has the form of the Complete Triangle.

The construction can be interpreted as follows. Circle 1 is 'square' — it simply fits comfortably into its own square. Circle 2 is bold: it ventures out to kiss Circle 1 beyond its own square. Circle 3 holds the two squares in balance. In doing so it produces the Complete (perfectly balanced) Triangle.

## 4. PROPERTIES OF THE TRIANGLE

If we drop a perpendicular CD from C to the base AB, the lengths of the sides form a geometric series of powers of r:

AB : BC : CA have lengths equal to the powers 0 : 1 : 2

CB : BD : DC have lengths equal to the powers 1 : 2 : 3

AC : CD : DA have lengths equal to the powers 2 : 3 : 4

The triangle can be successively subdivided, starting with the perpendicular DE from D to BC. The next stage will involve two perpendiculars — from D to AC and from E to DB. A stage of subdivision consists of dropping perpendiculars from the vertex of each of the larger triangles to the opposite side. At each stage the whole figure consists of only two basic triangles whose areas are related in the ratio of the Golden Mean.

The number of larger triangles at each stage forms a Fibonacci series. This is the series representing growth which is observed throughout the natural world (1, 2, 3, 5, 8, 13...) where each term is the sum of the two preceding terms. The same is true of the number of smaller triangles, one step behind, and the number of perpendiculars one step behind that.

Each line which is parallel to one side and joins points on the other two sides will be gradually filled by the perpendiculars, and no perpendicular will fall outside such a line. This process will continue indefinitely, and each line will be completed after a finite number of subdivisions. At any particular point the triangle is incomplete, but we can sense the way in which the lines will eventually join up. This 'lining up' of the triangles is a unique characteristic of the Complete Triangle.

## 5. RELEVANCE OF THE TRIANGLE

The point of all this is not to ascribe some magical powers to this triangle, but to convey a sense of a perfect balance between internal and external reality. It is a purely formal illustration which shows how endless vistas open up when the balance is exactly right. This example in the field of simple mathematics shows how imagination and proper proportion can open up a finite situation to endless integrated richness.

Ordinary right-angled triangles form uncoordinated patterns as the process of dropping perpendiculars is repeated. We can imagine an adjustable right-angled triangle (with variable angle and fixed hypotenuse) in which this process has been carried out a large number of times, with each set of perpendiculars lying beyond the previous one. This will give a jumble of lines which will remain until the angle is exactly that of the Complete Triangle. At this point the whole structure will spring into place, and the perfectly fitting subdivisions — each set forming a unique pattern — will dance away to infinity.

## 6. NOTE ON DIAGRAM ON BOOK COVER

The figure 'acts out' the resolution of the apparently absolute conflict between circles and squares by generating the 'Complete Triangle' based on the square root of the Golden Mean.

Circles symbolize love, squares symbolize logic. In each half of the diagram (left and right) there are two squares and three arcs of circles. One circle, centred at a corner of the large square, is careful and static, fitting exactly into the square. The other circle, centred at the middle of a side of the large square, is bold and dynamic, reaching out beyond its own square to kiss the first circle. Where it meets the full circle it creates a point which reconciles everything by producing triangles which fit in with each other in a continual dance as they are subdivided further and further. All three circles are necessary — static and dynamic are reconciled through their relationship to the whole.

The sides of the triangles all line up, but the intervals vary, and there are many lines which are still incomplete. This will always be true however much we subdivide the triangles. The balance is exact and yet does not feel rigidly formalized, even in such a formal field as geometry; it is simply 'right'. It illustrates the complete perfection of the deeply responsive middle way which is so especially espoused by Aristotle and Anglicanism.

The right half represents the outer world (World 1) and the left half represents the inner world (World 2). In some cases two triangles on the left correspond to one on the right, and in other cases there is a one-to-one correspondence. The shading for triangles in the inner world is generated at random (i.e. according to the choices that happen to be made). The shading for the outer world is generated by a formal method from the shading of the corresponding triangles on the left. This means there is a link via World 3 between World 1 and World 2. The central white triangle in each half symbolizes Christ, who is completely open to the light and links the two halves by his presence. There is no way in which this can be incorporated geometrically, but one can think of his love as 'longing' the triangles round to the angle which restores everything to wholeness.

The circle is the Whole, subjecting itself to the constraints of necessity (the squares). It also reminds us of the endless cycle of Hindu mythology. The pattern of black and white outside the triangles contains a hint of the yin-yang symbol of Chinese philosophy. The figure reveals fourfold form (the cross, with a white vertical and a black horizontal; the four slopes of the sides of the triangles — vertical, right, left, horizontal); duality in the relationship between smaller and large triangles on each side, between white and black, and between left and right sides; trinity in the shades, in the two-and-one of the corresponding triangles, in the three sizes of triangle, and the three circles in each half. At the very centre is the still point.

# INDEX

Words which occur too frequently to list are indicated by 'passim' ( = 'everywhere') followed by the total number of times they occur, in brackets. A few word-endings have been combined: eg. 'optimism' includes 'optimist'', and 'complementarity' includes 'complementary'.